The
Gym-Free
Fitness
Blueprint

BY KAUSTUBH M. KAISUKAR

Contents

Introduction

Conclusion
Your Fitness Journey

About the Author
kaisukarkaustubh385@gmail.com

ISBN: 9798300360672

Copyright Disclaimer

INTRODUCTION

In today's world, the idea of fitness is often tied to the gym—the clanging of weights, the rows of treadmills, and the strict routines designed to sculpt the perfect body. But what if I told you that you don't need a gym to be fit? What if I told you that fitness can be found in the simplest of movements, in the choices you make every day, and in embracing your body's natural ability to move and thrive?

Fitness isn't about equipment, fancy machines, or expensive memberships. It's about your [1]health, your energy, and your body's natural design to be strong, mobile, and resilient. The truth is, fitness is not a one-size-fits-all approach, nor does it have to be a rigid, structured routine. It can be as simple as taking the stairs instead of the elevator, stretching in the morning, or going for a walk in the park. Fitness can—and should—fit into your lifestyle seamlessly, whether you're a busy professional, a parent with limited time, or someone who simply prefers to avoid the hustle of the gym.

This book is for those who want to be active but aren't drawn to the idea of spending hours at a gym. It's for the person who believes that health and wellness don't have to come from a place of confinement or stress. It's for anyone who has felt overwhelmed by the pressure of fitting into society's narrow idea of what fitness looks like.

1

Here, we'll explore how you can achieve lasting fitness without stepping foot in a gym. Through bodyweight exercises, creative movement, outdoor activities, and a focus on overall well-being, we'll break down the barriers that make fitness seem complicated or unattainable. This isn't a book about extremes or drastic transformations—it's about finding balance, joy, and long-term health.

Fitness is a journey, not a destination. It's not about how much weight you can lift, how fast you can run, or how perfectly you can perform an exercise. It's about embracing your body's potential, making movement a regular part of your life, and, most importantly, finding joy in the process. When you move naturally and consistently, you not only get stronger, but you feel better, both physically and mentally.

In the following chapters, we'll uncover how to build sustainable habits, how to make fitness a part of your daily routine, and how to reclaim your health on your terms. You don't need a gym to live a strong, vibrant, and healthy life. All you need is the will to move, the knowledge to do so effectively, and the belief that fitness is for everyone, everywhere.

Let's get started.

CHAPTER 1

REDEFINING FITNESS

What is Fitness, Really?

For many, the word "fitness" conjures up images of chiselled abs, marathon runners, or sweaty gym-goers lifting weights. But fitness, in its truest sense, is much broader than aesthetics or performance. At its core, fitness is the state of being physically, mentally, and emotionally capable of meeting life's demands and challenges.

Physical fitness is about more than being able to run a mile or lift a certain amount of weight. It encompasses strength, endurance, flexibility, and balance—abilities that allow us to move through life with ease. However, mental and emotional fitness are just as vital. What's the point of having a strong body if your mind feels frazzled or your emotions are in turmoil?

In a holistic view, fitness is about thriving. It's the energy to chase after your kids without gasping for breath, the mental clarity to navigate your workday, and the emotional resilience to handle stress. By this definition, fitness extends far beyond the walls of a gym—it belongs wherever you are.

The Problem With Gym-Centric Fitness Culture Gyms, while popular, have unintentionally narrowed how society views fitness. The commercial fitness industry often equates health with gym memberships, specialised equipment, or the latest workout trends. This narrow view leads many to believe that if they can't afford a gym, don't have time to commute to one, or feel intimidated by the atmosphere, fitness isn't for them.

But the truth is, the human body is an adaptable, efficient machine that was designed to move. Long before gyms existed, humans stayed fit by walking, running, lifting, climbing, and engaging in everyday physical tasks. Our ancestors didn't need dumbbells to build strength or treadmills to run—they used what their environment provided. By reconnecting with this natural approach to movement, you can achieve a level of fitness that is both practical and sustainable.

Moreover, gym-based routines often isolate movements: a leg press for your quads, a bench press for your chest. While these exercises are effective, they don't always translate to functional strength—strength that helps you perform real-world tasks, like carrying groceries, gardening, or playing with your kids. Outside the gym, movements are more dynamic, engaging multiple muscle groups and mimicking the natural ways our bodies were meant to work.

Fitness as a Personal Journey

One of the most liberating truths about fitness is that it's deeply personal. There's no one-size-fits-all approach. Your fitness journey might involve long walks in the park, yoga on your living room floor, or bodyweight workouts in your backyard. The key is finding what works for you—activities that align with your goals, lifestyle, and preferences.

For example, someone who enjoys nature might find fulfilment in hiking or cycling on trails. A parent juggling work and kids might prefer short, high-intensity bodyweight workouts that can be done at home. What matters isn't the setting or the equipment but the consistency of effort and the joy you derive from the process.

Fitness should empower, not overwhelm. It's not about fitting into a mold or competing with others. It's about discovering what makes you feel strong, confident, and capable in your own skin.

Holistic Fitness: The Mind-Body Connection

Holistic fitness recognizes that the body, mind, and emotions are interconnected. When you engage in physical activity, it's not just your muscles that benefit—your brain and mood do too. Exercise releases endorphins, the feel-good chemicals that reduce stress and boost happiness. It sharpens your mental focus and improves memory. It even helps regulate sleep, a cornerstone of overall well-being.

Embracing fitness without the gym allows you to integrate mindfulness into your routine. Yoga, tai chi, or even a mindful walk in the woods can serve as both physical and mental workouts, calming your mind while strengthening your body. These practices emphasise being present in the moment, tuning into your breath, and listening to your body's signals—skills that can carry over into other areas of your life.

The Freedom of Gym-Free Fitness

The beauty of a gym-free fitness lifestyle is its freedom. You're not tied to specific hours, locations, or machines. You can move whenever and wherever you feel inspired—whether that's a few stretches in your kitchen while waiting for coffee to brew or a brisk walk around your neighbourhood after dinner.

Here are some examples of how you can embrace gym-free fitness in your everyday life:

1. Bodyweight Strength Training:

   - Push-ups, squats, planks, and lunges are highly effective and require no equipment.

   - These exercises can be modified to match your fitness level and gradually scaled as you improve.

2. Functional Movements:

   - Activities like carrying groceries, climbing stairs, or playing with your pets improve strength and endurance naturally.

3. Outdoor Activities:

   - From hiking to running, cycling to swimming, the outdoors offers endless opportunities to move your body while enjoying nature.

4. Movement Breaks:

   - Set a timer to stand, stretch, or do a quick set of exercises every hour if you work a sedentary job.

Debunking Myths About Gym-Free Fitness

Let's address a common myth: "You can't build serious strength or fitness without a gym." This simply isn't true. Bodyweight exercises, resistance bands, and other minimal equipment methods can build incredible strength, endurance, and flexibility. In fact, many athletes incorporate these methods into their training because they promote functional movement and injury prevention.

Another myth is that home workouts or outdoor activities aren't as effective as structured gym routines. The truth is, consistency trumps intensity. A few well-executed, intentional movements each day can yield significant results over time.

Taking the First Step

Redefining fitness starts with a mindset shift. Forget the idea that you need a perfect plan, expensive gear, or a gym membership to get started. All you need is the willingness to move. Begin by asking yourself these questions:

- What activities do I enjoy?

- How can I incorporate more movement into my day?

- What small, sustainable steps can I take toward my fitness goals?

Remember, fitness is a journey, not a destination. It's about building habits that enrich your life, not just your physique. So take a deep breath, step outside, and begin. Fitness is everywhere—you just have to find your rhythm.

CHAPTER 2

MINDSET FIRST: THE PSYCHOLOGY OF FITNESS

Introduction: The Mind-Body Connection

Fitness begins long before you lace up your shoes or hit your first push-up. It starts in your mind. Your thoughts, beliefs, and attitudes about exercise profoundly influence your ability to stay consistent and motivated. This chapter explores how to overcome mental barriers to fitness and cultivate a mindset that drives discipline and sustainable motivation.

Section 1: Overcoming Mental Barriers to Exercise

1.1 Common Mental Barriers

1. "I don't have time."

- Time is often the biggest perceived obstacle, but it's a matter of priorities. Most people can carve out 20-30 minutes daily by reassessing their schedules.

- Solution: Reframe exercise as a non-negotiable self-care practice, just like brushing your teeth.

2. " I'm too tired."

- Physical activity can feel daunting when you're fatigued, but exercise often energises rather than depletes you.

- Solution: Start with low-intensity exercises like stretching or walking to build momentum.

3. " I'm not fit enough to start."

- Many people feel intimidated by fitness, especially when comparing themselves to others.

- Solution: Focus on your unique journey. Remember, everyone starts somewhere.

4. "I lack the motivation."

- Motivation is fleeting; discipline is what sustains progress. Waiting to "feel" like exercising will often lead to inaction.

- Solution: Develop habits that make exercise automatic, removing the need for daily decisions.

1.2 Addressing Limiting Beliefs

1. Identify negative self-talk.

   - Examples: "I'm not athletic," or "I always quit." Recognize these as temporary narratives, not truths.

   - Practice: Replace them with affirmations like, "I am becoming stronger every day."

2. Reframe exercise as a privilege.

   - Shift your perspective: Movement is something your body can do, not something it must do.

3. Visualise success.

   - Imagine the energy, strength, and confidence you'll feel after sticking to your routine.

Section 2: Cultivating Discipline

2.1 The Power of Small Wins

- Discipline grows with small victories. Start with manageable tasks, such as a 5-minute walk or a single set of push-ups.

- Build momentum by celebrating these achievements, no matter how small.

2.2 Create a Ritual

- Habits thrive in routine. Link exercise to a specific time or activity, such as a morning stretch after waking or a short walk after lunch.

- Example: Treat your workout clothes as a trigger. Once you put them on, the likelihood of exercising increases.

2.3 Focus on Consistency Over Perfection

- It's better to show up imperfectly than not at all. A 10-minute workout is still progress.

- Remember, fitness is a marathon, not a sprint. Long-term results come from steady, consistent effort.

Section 3: Cultivating Motivation

3.1 Finding Your "Why"

- Motivation starts with purpose. Ask yourself:

  - Why do you want to be fit? Is it to feel stronger, play with your kids, or improve your mental health?

  - Write down your "why" and revisit it when motivation wanes.

3.2 Make It Enjoyable

- If exercise feels like a chore, you're less likely to stick with it.

  - Experiment with different activities until you find something you enjoy, whether it's dancing, yoga, or hiking.

- Create a motivating environment: music, podcasts, or even a favourite TV show during workouts.

3.3 Gamify Your Fitness

- Turn exercise into a challenge or game:

- Use apps or trackers to set goals (e.g., hitting 10,000 steps daily).

- Reward yourself for milestones, like completing 10 workouts in a month.

3.4 Seek Accountability

- Share your goals with a friend or join a fitness group. Accountability increases commitment.

- Social connections often make fitness more enjoyable.

Section 4: Managing Setbacks

4.1 Accept Imperfection

- Life happens, and missing a workout doesn't mean failure.

- Avoid the "all-or-nothing" mindset. One skipped day doesn't derail your progress; quitting altogether does.

4.2 Learn from Slip-Ups

- Reflect on why you missed a workout or lost motivation.

- Was your routine too ambitious? Did external stressors get in the way?

  - Adjust and keep moving forward.

4.3 Celebrate Resilience

- Every time you overcome a challenge, you build mental strength.

  - View obstacles as opportunities to grow, not reasons to quit.

Section 5: Building a Fitness Identity

5.1 See Yourself as a Fit Person

- Identity drives behavior. Begin to think of yourself as someone who values fitness.

  - Example: Instead of saying, "I'm trying to exercise," say, "I am someone who exercises."

5.2 Surround Yourself with Positive Influences

- Environment shapes habits. Surround yourself with people and resources that inspire a healthy lifestyle.

- Follow fitness accounts, join online communities, or read success stories.

5.3 Embrace the Journey

- Fitness is not a destination but a lifelong journey.

- Focus on progress, not perfection. The goal is to be better than you were yesterday.

Conclusion: A Strong Mind Builds a Strong Body

Your mind is the foundation of your fitness journey. By overcoming mental barriers, cultivating discipline, and finding sustainable sources of motivation, you can create lasting habits that lead to a healthier, more vibrant life. Remember, the hardest part is starting. Once you take that first step, momentum will carry you forward.

CHAPTER 3 : UNDERSTANDING YOUR "WHY"

Fitness journeys often begin with a burst of enthusiasm—perhaps fueled by the desire to look better, feel healthier, or accomplish a specific challenge. But as days turn into weeks, and initial excitement gives way to routine, staying consistent can become a struggle. This is where understanding your "why" becomes critical. It is the anchor that keeps you grounded, the compass that points you in the right direction when motivation falters.

The Power of Purpose in Fitness

Every journey begins with a purpose, and fitness is no exception. Your "why" is the reason you decide to lace up your sneakers, roll out your yoga mat, or simply get moving. It's deeply personal, unique to you, and goes beyond surface-level goals. For some, it might be the hope of being able to run around with their children without getting winded. For others, it could be the desire to reduce stress, manage chronic pain, or simply feel more energetic throughout the day.

When you define your purpose clearly, it creates a strong emotional connection to your fitness routine. This connection is what makes fitness not just another task on your to-do list, but a meaningful practice that aligns with your values and goals.

Moving Beyond Aesthetics

One of the most common reasons people start a fitness journey is to change their appearance—lose weight, tone up, or build muscle. While there's nothing wrong with aesthetic goals, they often lack the depth needed to sustain long-term commitment. Why? Because these goals are external and can be fleeting. Once you achieve a specific number on the scale or a desired look in the mirror, the question arises: what's next?

Shifting the focus to internal benefits—like feeling stronger, reducing stress, or improving mental clarity—creates a foundation for lifelong fitness. Internal goals tap into how exercise makes you feel rather than how it makes you look. This shift not only helps you stay consistent but also allows you to enjoy the process rather than focusing solely on the outcome.

Defining Personal Fitness Goals

The first step in defining your "why" is to identify what fitness truly means to you. Take some time to reflect on questions like:

- What do I want to achieve through fitness?

- How will being more active improve my life?

- What challenges am I facing that exercise can help address?

Write down your answers, and be as specific as possible. Instead of saying, "I want to be healthier," dig deeper. What does health mean to you? Is it the ability to climb stairs without feeling winded? Managing stress more effectively? Improving your sleep? The more specific your goals, the easier it is to create a plan that aligns with them.

Once you've identified your goals, break them into smaller, actionable steps. For example:

- Long-term goal: "I want to run a 5K in six months."

- Short-term goal: "I will start by jogging for 10 minutes three times a week."

Breaking goals into manageable chunks makes them less overwhelming and gives you a sense of accomplishment as you progress.

The Importance of Intention

Intention adds depth to your actions. It's the reason behind your effort, the "why" that keeps you going even on the days you'd rather hit snooze. When you exercise with intention, you're not just going through the motions; you're actively engaging with your body and mind to create a meaningful experience.

For example, let's say your goal is to improve your flexibility. Rather than mindlessly stretching because you "have to," approach each stretch with curiosity and focus. Pay attention to how your body feels, notice areas of tension, and celebrate even small improvements. This intentional approach transforms fitness from a chore into a practice of self-care and growth.

How to Stay Connected to Your "Why"

Life is full of distractions, and it's easy to lose sight of your original purpose. To stay connected to your "why," consider these strategies:

1. Write It Down

Keep a fitness journal or create a vision board with images and quotes that reflect your goals. Seeing your "why" visually can reinforce your commitment and remind you of the bigger picture.

2. Revisit and Adjust

Your goals and priorities may evolve over time, and that's okay. Periodically revisit your "why" to ensure it still resonates with you. If it doesn't, take the time to redefine it.

3. Celebrate Milestones

Acknowledge your progress, no matter how small. Each step you take toward your goal is a testament to your dedication and effort. Celebrating milestones reinforces your "why" and motivates you to keep going.

4. Find Accountability

Share your goals with a trusted friend, family member, or fitness community. Having someone to cheer you on or hold you accountable can strengthen your commitment.

Examples of a Strong "Why"

Here are some examples of meaningful "whys" that go beyond superficial goals:

- "I want to stay active so I can play with my grandchildren without pain."

- "Exercise helps me manage anxiety and feel more grounded."

- "I want to hike a mountain trail I've always dreamed of exploring."

- "Strength training makes me feel empowered and capable in my daily life."

Each of these reasons is deeply personal and tied to a specific outcome that enhances the individual's quality of life. They serve as a reminder of why fitness is worth the effort, even when motivation wanes.

From "Why" to Action

Once you've identified your "why," the next step is to turn it into action. Start by setting a consistent routine that aligns with your goals. Remember, consistency matters more than intensity. It's better to exercise for 10 minutes every day than to push yourself for an hour once a week and then give up.

As you move forward, stay flexible and forgiving. Life will inevitably throw curveballs, and there will be days when sticking to your routine feels impossible. On those days, reconnect with your "why." Remind yourself of the bigger picture and the long-term benefits of your efforts.

Conclusion

Understanding your "why" is the foundation of a sustainable fitness journey. It gives you clarity, purpose, and the resilience to keep going when the initial excitement fades. By focusing on deeply personal and meaningful goals, you can create a fitness routine that not only improves your physical health but also enhances your overall quality of life. So take the time to explore your "why." Once you've found it, hold onto it tightly—it's the key to unlocking your full potential.

CHAPTER 4

THE EVOLUTION OF MOVEMENT

Fitness, in its truest sense, has always been part of the human experience. Long before gyms became symbols of modern health, humans maintained physical strength, endurance, and agility through necessity, culture, and creativity. By tracing the historical roots of movement, we can uncover timeless practices that continue to be relevant and effective today.

Movement as Survival

For our ancient ancestors, movement wasn't optional—it was a matter of survival. Hunting, foraging, building shelters, and travelling long distances demanded physical strength and endurance. These natural movements—running, climbing, lifting, and throwing—shaped the bodies of early humans. Without formal exercises or fitness routines, their daily activities mirrored what we now call "functional fitness."

Anthropological studies suggest that hunter-gatherers were exceptionally fit by modern standards. They walked or ran long distances daily, climbed trees for fruit, and carried heavy loads of food or materials. These activities required a combination of strength, agility, and cardiovascular endurance. The term "use it or lose it" applied inherently to their lifestyle. If they didn't move, they didn't eat.

Ancient Civilizations and Organized Fitness

As human societies advanced, movement evolved beyond survival. Ancient civilizations began to formalise physical fitness practices, often linking them to cultural or spiritual beliefs. For example, the ancient Greeks and Romans were pioneers of structured physical training. In Greece, physical fitness was central to the concept of arete (virtue or excellence). The Olympic Games, founded in 776 BCE, showcased the Greeks' dedication to physical prowess and celebrated athletic ability as a mark of personal and societal greatness.

The Romans, too, emphasised physical training, particularly for military purposes. Roman soldiers engaged in rigorous training regimens, including marching, wrestling, and sword fighting. These activities were designed to prepare them for the physical demands of battle. While the Romans didn't have gyms as we know them today, their ludi (training schools) provided a space for combat and athletic preparation.

In ancient India, physical discipline was intertwined with spirituality. Yoga, which originated over 5,000 years ago, was not only a method of maintaining physical health but also a path to mental clarity and spiritual enlightenment. The postures, or asanas, strengthened the body while promoting flexibility and balance. Similarly, ancient Chinese practices like Tai Chi emphasised slow, deliberate movements that harmonised the body and mind.

Martial Arts: Movement as Skill and Discipline

Martial arts traditions from around the world demonstrate how movement evolved into an art form. In Asia, martial arts like Kung Fu, Karate, and Judo developed as both defensive techniques and methods of self-mastery. These practices required practitioners to build strength, flexibility, and precision. They also incorporated elements of mindfulness, teaching students to be present and focused.

In Africa, Capoeira emerged as a unique blend of martial art, dance, and acrobatics. Developed by enslaved Africans in Brazil, Capoeira was a form of resistance and a celebration of cultural identity. Its fluid, dance-like movements demanded agility, coordination, and strength, showcasing how physical expression could serve multiple purposes.

These ancient practices weren't just about building physical strength—they were about discipline, community, and connection to something greater than oneself. The movements were deeply embedded in cultural traditions, reflecting the values and struggles of the societies that created them.

The Rise of Callisthenics and Bodyweight Training

The term "callisthenics" comes from the Greek words kallos (beauty) and sthenos (strength), emphasising the aesthetic and functional aspects of bodyweight exercises. While the Greeks practised rudimentary forms of callisthenics, the formalisation of these exercises gained momentum in the 19th and 20th centuries.

Bodyweight exercises, such as push-ups, pull-ups, and squats, became a cornerstone of physical fitness training due to their accessibility and effectiveness. Soldiers in various militaries used callisthenics to build strength and endurance without needing equipment. These exercises mimic natural movements, making them highly functional for real-life scenarios.

The beauty of callisthenics lies in its adaptability. A beginner can start with modified versions of exercises, such as push-ups on the knees, while advanced practitioners can progress to feats like one-arm push-ups or handstands. This scalability has ensured its lasting appeal across cultures and generations.

The Industrial Era and Fitness Decline

The industrial revolution marked a turning point in human movement. As machines took over manual labour, many people transitioned to sedentary lifestyles. The physical demands of daily life decreased, leading to a decline in natural fitness levels. However, this shift also sparked the creation of modern fitness movements.

In the 19th century, European and American fitness pioneers began advocating for structured exercise routines. Figures like Friedrich Ludwig Jahn in Germany promoted gymnastics as a way to build strength and discipline. Similarly, the YMCA, founded in the mid-19th century, encouraged physical activity as part of a holistic approach to well-being.

While these movements laid the groundwork for the fitness industry, they also highlighted a fundamental truth: humans need to move to thrive. The gym became a solution to the growing problem of inactivity, but it wasn't the only one.

Ancient Practices in Modern Times

Many ancient practices remain relevant because they align with the body's natural mechanics. Yoga, for instance, has experienced a global renaissance, with millions embracing it for its physical, mental, and emotional benefits. Modern yoga studios may look different from ancient ashrams, but the core principles remain the same: balance, flexibility, and mindfulness.

Similarly, martial arts continue to thrive as both a sport and a form of self-defense. Practices like Brazilian Jiu-Jitsu, Muay Thai, and Krav Maga combine ancient techniques with modern training methodologies, demonstrating the enduring value of these disciplines.

Calisthenics has also made a comeback, particularly in urban environments where public parks feature outdoor fitness stations. Social media has fueled interest in bodyweight training, with influencers showcasing advanced moves like muscle-ups and human flags.

Lessons from the Past

The evolution of movement teaches us that fitness doesn't require expensive equipment or a gym membership. The most effective exercises are often the simplest—movements that use the body as its own tool. Ancient practices remind us that fitness is about more than aesthetics; it's about functionality, resilience, and harmony.

By incorporating elements of yoga, martial arts, and callisthenics into our routines, we can tap into centuries of wisdom. These practices not only build strength and endurance but also foster mental clarity and a deeper connection to our bodies. Whether we're practising yoga in a quiet room, sparring with a partner, or performing pull-ups in a park, we're participating in a tradition that spans generations.

Fitness is not a modern invention; it's a human necessity. By returning to the roots of movement, we can rediscover a simpler, more holistic approach to health and well-being—one that's accessible to everyone, regardless of age, background, or fitness level.

CHAPTER 5

THE SCIENCE OF FUNCTIONAL FITNESS

Functional fitness is a term often used in modern fitness circles, but its principles are as old as humanity itself. At its core, functional fitness is about training your body to perform everyday activities with ease and efficiency. It emphasises movements that mimic real-life actions, such as squatting, lifting, pushing, pulling, and twisting. These exercises build strength, improve balance, enhance mobility, and develop endurance, all of which are crucial for a healthier and more resilient body.

What is Functional Fitness?

The idea behind functional fitness is simple: train your body to handle daily tasks more effectively. Unlike traditional weightlifting or machine-based gym workouts, functional exercises engage multiple muscle groups simultaneously and often involve movements performed in multiple planes of motion. For example, a squat combined with a rotation simulates bending down to pick up a heavy object and turning to place it elsewhere—a common action in everyday life.

Functional fitness isn't about isolating muscles for aesthetic purposes. Instead, it focuses on building a body that works harmoniously, making you better equipped to handle life's physical demands. This type of training improves coordination, posture, and balance while reducing the risk of injuries.

Understanding Natural Movement

Human bodies are designed for movement patterns that have evolved over thousands of years. Early humans didn't have treadmills or weight machines—they climbed, jumped, carried, ran, and balanced as part of their survival. These primal movements form the foundation of functional fitness, which seeks to restore and optimize these natural patterns.

Examples of natural movement include:

- Squatting: Sitting down and standing up, picking up objects, or gardening.

- Lunging: Walking uphill, stepping into a car, or navigating uneven terrain.

- Pulling and Pushing: Opening heavy doors, carrying groceries, or moving furniture.

- Rotating: Turning to grab something behind you or twisting to throw an object.

- Balancing: Walking on uneven surfaces or standing while carrying something.

Incorporating exercises that mimic these movements can improve not only your physical performance but also your quality of life.

Benefits of Functional Fitness

Functional fitness provides numerous benefits, making it an excellent option for people of all ages and fitness levels. Here's how it supports everyday life:

1. Improved Mobility

Mobility is the ability to move freely and efficiently through a full range of motion. Functional exercises enhance joint flexibility and muscle elasticity, making it easier to perform tasks like bending, reaching, and stretching. Better mobility also reduces stiffness and the likelihood of injury during physical activities.

2. Increased Strength

Strength isn't just about lifting heavy weights; it's about having the power to move your body and external objects effectively. Functional exercises like squats, push-ups, and lunges develop strength that translates into real-world applications, such as carrying groceries, climbing stairs, or playing with children.

3. Enhanced Endurance

Everyday life requires sustained energy. Whether you're on your feet all day at work or chasing after kids, functional fitness helps improve cardiovascular health and muscular endurance, ensuring you can keep up with life's demands.

4. Better Balance and Coordination

Many functional exercises challenge your stability, forcing you to engage your core and small stabilizing muscles. This improves balance and coordination, which are essential for activities like walking on uneven surfaces or carrying heavy loads without falling.

5. Injury Prevention

Functional training focuses on building a strong core, improving posture, and correcting imbalances between muscle groups. This reduces strain on joints and ligaments, lowering the risk of injuries in daily activities.

6. Boosted Confidence in Daily Activities

Functional fitness prepares your body for everyday tasks, making you feel more capable and confident. Whether it's lifting a heavy box or keeping up with an energetic pet, you'll notice an improvement in how you move through life.

Key Functional Exercises

Here are some essential functional fitness exercises and the natural movements they mimic:

- Squats

Squats are fundamental to sitting, standing, and lifting. They work the glutes, hamstrings, quadriceps, and core. Variations like goblet squats or adding a rotation engage more muscles and mimic lifting and twisting motions.

- Lunges

Lunges replicate stepping and help build strength in the legs and hips. They also improve balance and coordination, especially when done with added challenges like weights or unstable surfaces.

- Push-Ups

Push-ups strengthen the chest, shoulders, arms, and core while mimicking the motion of pushing objects. They're versatile and can be modified for different fitness levels.

- Pulls and Rows

Exercises like pull-ups or resistance band rows develop the pulling muscles in your back, biceps, and shoulders. These movements are essential for tasks like pulling a heavy door open or lifting objects toward you.

- Planks

Planks strengthen the core, which is central to nearly every movement. A strong core improves posture, reduces back pain, and enhances overall stability.

- Farmer's Carry

Carrying weights in each hand mimics carrying groceries, luggage, or other heavy items. It works the grip, arms, shoulders, and core while improving stability.

- Rotational Movements

Exercises like woodchoppers or Russian twists simulate the twisting motions used in sports and daily activities, such as reaching for something on a shelf or throwing a ball.

How to Incorporate Functional Fitness Into Your Routine

Functional fitness can be integrated into your daily life with minimal equipment. Start with bodyweight exercises, then progress to incorporating resistance bands, dumbbells, or even household items like water bottles or heavy books. Here are a few tips for building a functional fitness routine:

- Warm-Up: Always start with a dynamic warm-up to prepare your body for movement. Include exercises like arm circles, leg swings, and cat-cow stretches.

- Combine Movements: Create compound exercises by combining two or more motions. For example, try a squat-to-press or a lunge with a twist.

- Focus on Quality Over Quantity: Perform each movement with proper form to avoid injury and maximise benefits.

- Progress Gradually: Increase the intensity, duration, or complexity of exercises as you gain strength and confidence.

Functional Fitness for All Ages

One of the most significant advantages of functional fitness is its adaptability. Whether you're a young adult, a senior, or somewhere in between, functional exercises can be scaled to suit your needs. Older adults, for example, benefit from these exercises as they help maintain independence and reduce the risk of falls. Younger individuals can use functional fitness to enhance athletic performance or prepare for physically demanding jobs.

Final Thoughts

Functional fitness is a practical and effective approach to staying fit and healthy. By focusing on natural movements that mirror everyday activities, it prepares your body to handle life's physical demands with ease and efficiency. As you incorporate functional exercises into your routine, you'll not only see improvements in strength, endurance, and mobility but also experience greater confidence in your ability to move through life with power and grace.

CHAPTER 6

THE ESSENTIAL COMPONENTS OF FITNESSs

Introduction: Building Blocks of a Healthy Body

Imagine your body as a multi-faceted machine, each part playing a critical role in helping you move, lift, stretch, and recover. To maintain this machine, you need to focus on more than just one element of fitness. Strength without flexibility can lead to stiffness. Endurance without balance might leave you prone to injuries. True fitness is holistic—it's about building a body that is not only strong but also supple, resilient, and agile.

This chapter breaks down the four essential components of fitness—strength, flexibility, endurance, and balance—and offers guidance on how to weave them into a well-rounded workout routine that doesn't require a gym.

1. Strength: Building a Strong Foundation

Strength is the cornerstone of fitness. It enables you to carry groceries, lift furniture, and perform daily tasks with ease. Strong muscles also support your bones, reducing the risk of injuries and improving posture.

Key Benefits of Strength Training:

- Increases muscle mass, which boosts metabolism.

- Protects joints and improves bone density.

- Enhances athletic performance and functional movement.

Strength Without a Gym:

You don't need weights to build strength. Your body is your best tool. Bodyweight exercises like push-ups, squats, lunges, and planks are incredibly effective. For added resistance, try resistance bands or household items like water jugs.

Sample Strength Routine:

- Push-ups: 3 sets of 10–15 reps.

- Bodyweight squats: 3 sets of 15–20 reps.

- Plank hold: 3 sets of 30–60 seconds.

- Resistance band rows (using a door anchor): 3 sets of 12–15 reps.

2. Flexibility: Moving Freely and Easily

Flexibility often takes a backseat to strength and endurance, but it's equally important. It's what allows you to bend, twist, and stretch without pain or restriction. A lack of flexibility can lead to poor posture, muscle imbalances, and injuries.

Key Benefits of Flexibility Training:

- Improves range of motion in joints.

- Reduces muscle tightness and soreness.

- Enhances coordination and balance.

Flexibility Without a Gym:

Stretching routines or yoga sessions are perfect for improving flexibility. You can do these at home, in a park, or even during a break at work.

Sample Flexibility Routine:

- Forward fold (hamstring stretch): Hold for 20–30 seconds.

- Cat-cow stretch (spinal mobility): Perform for 1–2 minutes.

- Butterfly stretch (inner thighs): Hold for 20–30 seconds.

- Downward dog (full-body stretch): Hold for 30 seconds, repeat 3 times.

3. Endurance: The Heart of Fitness

Endurance refers to your ability to sustain physical activity over time, whether it's a brisk walk, a swim, or a full day of errands. It's a measure of your cardiovascular and muscular stamina. A strong heart and lungs are critical for long-term health.

Key Benefits of Endurance Training:

- Strengthens the heart and improves circulation.

- Increases energy levels by improving oxygen delivery.

- Supports weight management through calorie burn.

Endurance Without a Gym:

Cardio doesn't have to involve a treadmill. Walking, jogging, biking, or even dancing are great ways to boost endurance. Interval training—alternating bursts of intense effort with rest—is particularly effective and can be done anywhere.

Sample Endurance Routine:

- Brisk walk or jog: 20–30 minutes.

- High knees (in place): 3 sets of 30 seconds.

- Stair climbing: 5–10 minutes.

- Jumping jacks: 3 sets of 30 seconds.

4. Balance: Staying Steady and Controlled

Balance is often overlooked, yet it's a vital component of fitness. It's what keeps you steady on your feet, prevents falls, and enhances coordination. Balance training is especially important as we age, but it benefits people of all ages.

Key Benefits of Balance Training:

- Improves proprioception (awareness of body position in space).

- Reduces risk of falls and injuries.

- Enhances performance in sports and daily activities.

Balance Without a Gym:

Simple exercises like standing on one leg, walking heel-to-toe, or practicing yoga poses like the tree pose can help. Balance training doesn't require any equipment and can be done anywhere.

Sample Balance Routine:

- Single-leg stand: Hold for 30 seconds per leg.

- Heel-to-toe walk: 2–3 minutes.

- Tree pose: Hold for 30 seconds per side.

- Bosu ball alternative: Use a pillow or unstable surface for added challenge.

5. Designing a Well-Rounded Workout Routine

Creating a routine that includes all four components doesn't have to be complicated. Here's how to structure your week for a balanced approach:

Sample Weekly Plan:

- Monday: Strength (30 minutes) + flexibility (10 minutes).

- Tuesday: Endurance (30 minutes).

- Wednesday: Rest or active recovery (light stretching or yoga).

- Thursday: Strength (30 minutes) + balance (10 minutes).

- Friday: Endurance (30 minutes).

- Saturday: Combined session (15 minutes of strength, 15 minutes of cardio, 10 minutes of flexibility).

- Sunday: Rest or a recreational activity (e.g., hiking or swimming).

Tips for Staying Consistent:

1. Start Small: If you're new to fitness, aim for 10–15 minutes per session and gradually increase duration.

2. Mix It Up: Avoid monotony by alternating activities, locations, and routines.

3. Listen to Your Body: Take rest days when needed, especially if you feel sore or fatigued.

6. Integrating Fitness Into Daily Life

Fitness doesn't have to feel like a chore. Incorporate these components into your everyday life:

- Take the stairs instead of the elevator (endurance).

- Stretch while watching TV (flexibility).

- Practice balance by standing on one leg while brushing your teeth.

- Carry heavy grocery bags (strength).

Conclusion: The Symbiosis of Fitness Components

Strength, flexibility, endurance, and balance are interconnected. Neglecting one can create imbalances that hinder overall fitness. By focusing on all four components, you'll build a body that's not only fit but also functional and resilient. Whether you're at home, at a park, or traveling, this holistic approach ensures you're prepared for whatever life throws your way.

CHAPTER 7

DESIGNING A GYM-FREE ROUTINE

Adapting to Different Lifestyles and Time Constraints

One of the most common reasons people feel they can't maintain a consistent fitness routine is because they believe they don't have enough time. Whether you have a busy work schedule, family commitments, or a packed social life, the key to designing a gym-free routine is adaptability. Fitness should fit seamlessly into your lifestyle, not be a burden that feels like an extra obligation.

The beauty of working out without the gym is that you're not restricted by set hours, travel time, or expensive memberships. You have the flexibility to exercise whenever and wherever you want, whether it's in the morning before work, during a lunch break, or in the evening after dinner. The trick is to plan your workouts based on your available time, physical capacity, and the space around you.

Step 1: Assess Your Current Schedule

Before diving into your workout routine, take a week to observe your schedule. Are there pockets of time throughout the day where you could fit in exercise, even if it's just for 10 or 20 minutes? You don't need hours on end to get fit. The goal is to use your available time efficiently. For example:

- Busy Morning Routine: Consider a 10-minute bodyweight circuit to kickstart your day. Simple exercises like squats, push-ups, and jumping jacks will get your heart rate up and set a positive tone for the day.

- Lunch Breaks: If you have a longer break, take 30 minutes to go for a brisk walk or cycle. You can also perform a quick full-body workout with resistance bands or dumbbells.

- Evening Wind-Down: Stretching or doing yoga for 20 minutes before bed can help reduce stress and improve sleep.

Step 2: Identify Your Fitness Level

Once you've determined where and when to fit exercise in your schedule, it's time to tailor your workout routine based on your fitness level. Whether you're a beginner, intermediate, or advanced, it's important to respect your body's current capabilities and challenge it progressively.

1. Beginners:

If you're just starting, the goal should be to establish a habit. Your body will need time to adjust to regular exercise, and your focus should be on building a foundation of strength, endurance, and flexibility. For beginners, simplicity is key.

- Frequency: Aim for 3-4 workouts per week.

- Duration: Start with 20-30 minutes per session.

- Focus: A mix of bodyweight exercises (like squats, lunges, push-ups), walking, and flexibility work (like stretching or beginner yoga).

2. Intermediate:

If you have some experience with exercise, you can start incorporating more variety and intensity into your routine. You might be ready for a combination of strength training, cardio, and flexibility, with a greater focus on intensity.

   - Frequency: 4-5 workouts per week.

   - Duration: 30-45 minutes per session.

   - Focus: A balanced mix of bodyweight exercises, resistance bands or light dumbbells, and outdoor activities (running, cycling, or hiking).

3. Advanced:

For more seasoned fitness enthusiasts, the goal is to push your body to the next level. You're likely focusing on either strength, endurance, or mobility, and incorporating higher-intensity exercises, complex movements, and longer sessions.

   - Frequency: 5-6 workouts per week.

   - Duration: 45-60 minutes per session.

- Focus: More intense bodyweight exercises, weighted routines, plyometrics, HIIT (High-Intensity Interval Training), or outdoor endurance activities.

Step 3: Weekly Plans for All Levels

Now that you have a clear understanding of your fitness level and available time, here's how you can structure your weekly gym-free workout routine. Remember, consistency is more important than perfection. A well-rounded plan should include strength training, cardiovascular work, and flexibility.

Beginner Routine:

- Monday: Full Body Strength Circuit (30 minutes)

  - Warm-up: 5-10 minutes of light cardio (jogging in place, jumping jacks)

  - Circuit (3 rounds):

    - 10 Squats

    - 10 Push-ups (modified if necessary)

    - 15-second plank

- 10 Glute bridges

- 15 Jumping jacks

- Cool-down: 5 minutes of stretching

- Wednesday: Active Recovery (30 minutes)

  - Light stretching or beginner yoga. Focus on flexibility and mobility.

- Friday: Walk or Low-Impact Cardio (30 minutes)

  - Go for a brisk walk or cycle around your neighborhood. Try to increase your pace slightly every week to improve endurance.

- Sunday: Flexibility and Relaxation (20 minutes)
  - Focus on full-body stretches or gentle yoga.

Intermediate Routine:

- Monday: Bodyweight Strength Circuit (40 minutes)

- Warm-up: 5-10 minutes of light cardio (jump rope, high knees)

  - Circuit (4 rounds):

    - 15 Squats

    - 12 Push-ups

    - 20 Walking lunges (each leg)

    - 30-second plank

    - 15 Burpees

  - Cool-down: 5 minutes of stretching

- Tuesday: Cardio (35-40 minutes)

  - Running, cycling, or hiking. Gradually increase your pace or distance each week.

- Thursday: Resistance Training (40 minutes)

  - Using resistance bands or dumbbells, do exercises such as:

    - 12-15 Dumbbell squats

    - 12-15 Dumbbell rows

- 12-15 Overhead press (using dumbbells or resistance bands)

    - 15 Bicep curls

  - Cool-down: Stretch or foam roll.

- Saturday: HIIT Workout (20-30 minutes)

  - Warm-up: 5 minutes of light cardio

  - HIIT circuit (repeat 3-4 times):

    - 30 seconds Jump squats

    - 30 seconds Push-ups

    - 30 seconds Mountain climbers

    - 30 seconds Burpees

    - 1-minute rest

  - Cool-down: 5 minutes of stretching

Advanced Routine:

- Monday: Strength and Plyometrics (50 minutes)

- Warm-up: 5-10 minutes of light cardio (jump rope, high knees)

  - Circuit (4 rounds):

    - 20 Jump squats

    - 15 Push-ups (add variations like diamond or incline)

    - 20 Walking lunges with knee drive

    - 1-minute plank hold

    - 15 Burpees

  - Cool-down: 5 minutes of deep stretching

- Tuesday: Long Cardio (45-60 minutes)

  - Run, bike, or hike at a moderate pace. This is a low-to-moderate intensity session to build endurance.

- Thursday: Full Body Strength (45-50 minutes)

  - Incorporate resistance bands, dumbbells, and bodyweight exercises to target all major muscle groups:

    - 15 Deadlifts (with weights or resistance bands)

    - 15 Rows

    - 15 Push-ups

- 20 Squats

- Cool-down: Stretching or foam rolling.

- Saturday: HIIT or Outdoor Challenge (40 minutes)

- Choose either a HIIT workout or an outdoor activity like stair climbing, sprints, or circuit training in the park.

Step 4: Consistency and Flexibility

Designing a gym-free routine isn't just about creating a plan and sticking to it rigidly—it's about consistency and flexibility. Life happens, and sometimes your schedule might not go as planned. That's okay! The beauty of working out outside of the gym is the ability to adapt. If you miss a workout, simply adjust your plan and get back at it the next day. The most important part is maintaining a habit that's sustainable for you.

By creating a personalized gym-free routine that adapts to your time constraints, lifestyle, and fitness level, you set yourself up for success. The goal is to make exercise an integral part of your life, regardless of whether you have access to a gym. With consistency, a bit of creativity, and an adaptable mindset, you can achieve your fitness goals without stepping foot in a gym.

CHAPTER 8

FITNESS ANYWHERE: MAKING ANY SPACE WORK

One of the most beautiful aspects of fitness is that it doesn't require an expansive gym or a state-of-the-art facility. Whether you live in a cramped apartment, have a spacious backyard, or enjoy the open air of a nearby park, your workout zone is wherever you decide to create it. The key to maintaining fitness outside of the gym is learning how to use what you have around you—whether that's your living room floor, a small corner in your bedroom, or a patch of grass in a local park.

Transforming Your Living Room Into a Fitness Space

You don't need a fancy home gym setup to stay in shape. One of the easiest and most accessible workout spaces is the very room you're in right now. Whether it's your living room, bedroom, or a multipurpose space, it can quickly become your personal fitness zone.

1. Clear the Space

The first step is simple: create space. If your living room is filled with furniture, books, or toys, spend a few minutes pushing things to the side. Move a coffee table out of the way or push the sofa slightly to the side if possible. A few feet of open space is all you need for most bodyweight exercises. Don't be intimidated by clutter; it's just a matter of creating a dedicated area for movement. Even a 6-foot by 6-foot space can be enough for most workouts.

2. Use Household Items as Equipment

If you don't have any fitness equipment, don't worry—household items can work wonders in a pinch. Use a sturdy chair or couch for elevated push-ups, tricep dips, or step-ups. A thick towel can serve as a yoga mat, and a backpack filled with books can act as a weighted vest for squats or lunges. For resistance training, consider using water bottles, laundry detergent bottles, or canned goods as makeshift dumbbells.

3. Incorporate Cardio

Cardio doesn't have to involve fancy machines. Jump rope in your living room (just be mindful of the space around you), or perform high-intensity interval training (HIIT) exercises like burpees, mountain climbers, or jumping jacks. These exercises are incredibly effective for burning fat and building endurance, and they require no special equipment.

Turning Your Backyard Into a Fitness Sanctuary

If you're lucky enough to have outdoor space, your backyard can become a fitness paradise, combining fresh air, natural beauty, and the potential for a full-body workout. The versatility of outdoor spaces offers more freedom to experiment and move, plus the benefits of sunshine and nature's tranquility.

1. Using Nature as Your Gym

Your backyard is full of potential fitness equipment. Trees, fences, and benches can serve as tools for your workouts. Try hanging a pull-up bar on a sturdy tree branch, or use a fence to practice incline push-ups. You can also practice agility drills, jump rope, or sprint intervals on a grassy patch. Set up an obstacle course for a fun, heart-pumping workout. Nature itself can provide great resistance training—think of running up hills, climbing trees, or pushing against resistance with wind or uneven surfaces.

2. Minimal Equipment for Maximum Impact

Even without elaborate gym equipment, you can create a well-rounded workout in your backyard. A pair of dumbbells, a kettlebell, or a resistance band can go a long way. These tools are relatively inexpensive, easy to store, and offer a variety of exercises that challenge different muscle groups. If you don't want to purchase any equipment, simply use your body's weight in exercises like squats, lunges, push-ups, and planks, which require no external tools.

3. The Importance of Stretching Outdoors

Stretching in the open air can enhance your flexibility while boosting your mood. Use the open space to practice yoga or Pilates, or follow a guided stretching routine to improve flexibility and reduce muscle tightness. The calming effect of being outside can also aid in relaxation, helping you recover mentally and physically after a workout.

Creating a Fitness Routine for Small Spaces

For those who live in apartments or have limited space, finding ways to work out in a smaller area might feel like a challenge. But even in the smallest of rooms, you can perform an effective workout with minimal equipment. Small spaces are ideal for bodyweight exercises, yoga, Pilates, or dance.

1. Utilize Vertical Space

When floor space is limited, look up! Pull-ups, chin-ups, and rows can all be performed with a sturdy doorframe bar or a doorway attachment. If you're short on space, consider using resistance bands, which are compact, portable, and provide versatile resistance for upper body, lower body, and core exercises.

2. Compact Equipment

Investing in compact fitness equipment can also be a game-changer for small spaces. Resistance bands, dumbbells, or kettlebells are easy to store and don't take up much room. A yoga mat or exercise ball can easily be rolled up and put away after each session, freeing up space for other activities. Additionally, many fitness tools like jump ropes, balance boards, and sliders are small but highly effective.

3. Focus on Bodyweight Movements

When space is tight, bodyweight exercises are your best friend. You can perform push-ups, squats, lunges, planks, and burpees without taking up much space. Circuits of bodyweight exercises can elevate your heart rate, build strength, and increase flexibility, all while requiring only the space you have at hand. Using small movements like wall sits or tabletop exercises is also great for working specific muscles without moving around much.

Fitness in the Park: Expanding Your Workout Horizons

Parks are one of the best places to work out without a gym. Not only do they provide ample open space, but they also offer access to free resources like walking trails, hills, and sometimes even fitness stations.

1. Nature's Obstacles

Parks can offer some of the best tools for functional fitness. You can run on trails, climb hills, or use park benches for step-ups, tricep dips, and Bulgarian split squats. Look for structures like low walls or fences that can act as bars for stretching or bodyweight rows. The environment offers variety that's missing in traditional gyms—no two workouts need to be the same!

2. Social and Mental Benefits

Exercising in a park can have social benefits, too. If you're looking to meet like-minded individuals or just want a change of scenery, consider joining outdoor fitness groups, participating in park runs, or practicing yoga in the open air. The fresh air and change of environment can also help improve your mental well-being, giving you a break from the stress of indoor spaces.

3. Outdoor Cardio

Many parks have tracks or long paths perfect for jogging or cycling. Combine your outdoor runs with bodyweight strength exercises like lunges, squats, and push-ups along the way. A simple run-walk routine paired with bodyweight exercises can provide a full-body workout while benefiting from the healing power of nature.

Conclusion

Fitness doesn't have to be confined to the gym, and it certainly doesn't require a large amount of space or expensive equipment. Your living room, backyard, or even a nearby park can be transformed into a workout zone with just a little creativity. By leveraging the space you have and using minimal equipment, you can achieve your fitness goals and enjoy a flexible, sustainable workout routine that fits into your lifestyle. The possibilities are endless—no gym required.

CHAPTER 9

BODYWEIGHT EXERCISES: YOUR BUILT-IN GYM

When it comes to building strength, endurance, and flexibility without stepping foot inside a gym, bodyweight exercises are your best friend. These exercises don't require fancy equipment or large spaces, yet they can transform your body into a powerhouse of functional strength. Push-ups, planks, squats, lunges, and others offer versatile options that target multiple muscle groups simultaneously. Whether you're a beginner or an advanced athlete, bodyweight exercises can be adjusted to suit your fitness level.

Push-ups: The Classic Upper Body Strengthener

Push-ups are a fundamental exercise that engages the chest, shoulders, arms, and core. They're an excellent bodyweight exercise because they require no equipment and can be modified for any fitness level.

Basic Push-ups:

Start by lying face down on the floor, placing your hands shoulder-width apart. As you press through your palms, keep your body in a straight line from head to heels, lowering yourself until your chest nearly touches the ground. Push back up to the starting position. This engages the pectoral muscles, triceps, and deltoids, with stabilization from the core.

Progression:

- Knee Push-ups: For beginners, start with your knees on the floor to reduce the amount of weight you're pushing up. This allows you to build strength while maintaining good form.

- Incline Push-ups: Place your hands on a raised surface like a bench or countertop. This will reduce the difficulty, allowing you to master the movement before progressing.

Advanced Variation:

- Archer Push-ups: A more challenging variation where one arm does the majority of the work, and the other extends out to the side. This challenges stability and strength.

- Decline Push-ups: Place your feet on a raised surface (such as a bench or step) to increase the intensity and target the upper chest and shoulders more.

Planks: Core Stability and Strength

Planks are perhaps the most effective exercise to build core strength, helping to stabilize your body during almost every movement. A strong core is essential for posture, balance, and overall functional strength.

Basic Plank:

Start in a forearm plank position. Your elbows should be directly under your shoulders, your body in a straight line from head to heels, and your core engaged. Keep your glutes and legs tight, ensuring your back doesn't sag. Hold this position for as long as you can while maintaining good form.

Progression:

- Knee Plank: If holding a full plank is too challenging, start by lowering your knees to the ground, ensuring your body remains in a straight line from your knees to your head.

Advanced Variation:

- Side Plank: Lie on your side, supporting your body with one forearm, and stack your feet. The side plank challenges the obliques and helps improve rotational strength. Hold for as long as you can before switching sides.

- Plank with Shoulder Taps: Start in the high plank position (hands on the floor). While keeping your hips stable, alternate tapping your opposite hand to the opposite shoulder. This adds a challenge to the core while engaging your upper body.

Squats: Lower Body Power

Squats are a powerhouse movement that works the quads, hamstrings, glutes, and core. It's a functional movement that mimics actions we perform every day, such as sitting, standing, and lifting.

Basic Squat:

Stand with your feet shoulder-width apart. Keep your chest upright and push your hips back as if sitting into a chair. Lower yourself until your thighs are parallel to the ground, making sure your knees stay behind your toes. Press through your heels to return to standing.

Progression:

- Box Squats: Use a sturdy box, chair, or bench to sit back onto. This variation helps you learn the correct movement pattern by allowing you to touch the surface and push back up.

Advanced Variation:

- Pistol Squat: A single-leg squat where one leg is extended straight in front of you while you squat down on the other leg. This requires significant balance, flexibility, and strength.

- Jump Squats: Add an explosive element by jumping as you rise from the squat position. This increases the intensity and helps build power in the legs.

Lunges: Strength and Stability

Lunges are another fantastic lower-body exercise that targets the quadriceps, hamstrings, glutes, and stabilizing muscles of the core. The movement involves stepping forward and lowering your body, which challenges your balance and coordination.

Basic Lunge:

Stand upright, feet together. Step forward with one foot, bending both knees to lower your hips toward the ground. The back knee should hover just above the floor, and the front knee should stay in line with the ankle (not extending past the toes). Push through the front heel to return to the standing position, and repeat with the opposite leg.

Progression:

- Reverse Lunges: Step backward instead of forward. This reduces the strain on the knees and may feel more stable for beginners.

- Static Lunges: Start with one foot forward and the other behind you. Lower your body into a lunge and then rise, without stepping forward or backward. This allows you to focus more on controlled movement.

Advanced Variation:

- Jumping Lunges: In a lunge position, jump and switch legs mid-air, landing in a lunge with the opposite leg forward. This adds cardiovascular intensity and explosive power.

- Bulgarian Split Squats: Place one foot on a bench or elevated surface behind you and perform a lunge. The increased range of motion targets the quads more intensely.

Burpees: Full-Body Power

While not part of the basic movements like push-ups or squats, burpees are a dynamic, high-intensity exercise that can quickly elevate your heart rate, improve cardiovascular fitness, and build muscle endurance.

Basic Burpee:

Start by standing upright. Drop into a squat position, placing your hands on the floor, and kick your feet back into a plank. Quickly return your feet to your hands, then explode upwards into a jump. Repeat.

Progression:

- Half Burpees: Skip the jump at the top and focus on the plank-to-squat movement. This reduces the intensity while still providing a great workout.

Advanced Variation:

- Chest-to-Floor Burpees: Lower yourself fully to the ground during the plank portion, making contact with your chest before pushing back up. This variation increases the time under tension and challenges your upper body strength.

Conclusion: Mastering Bodyweight Movements

Bodyweight exercises are not only effective but are also versatile and scalable for all fitness levels. Whether you're just starting or you're looking to push yourself with more advanced variations, there is a bodyweight movement to suit your goals.

The beauty of bodyweight training lies in its simplicity and accessibility—no gym, no fancy equipment, just your body and the ground beneath you. With consistent practice, you'll notice improvements in strength, endurance, balance, and mobility, all of which will translate into better overall fitness and a healthier lifestyle.

By incorporating these exercises into your routine, you'll have the tools to build a full-body workout that can be done anywhere, anytime. Stay committed, and remember, progress is built one push-up, one squat, and one plank at a time.

CHAPTER 10

FUNCTIONAL MOVEMENTS FOR EVERYDAY STRENGTH

In the fast-paced modern world, many of us sit behind desks, commute in cars, and spend hours on devices. Yet, despite this sedentary lifestyle, our bodies are designed for movement. Functional movements, which are exercises that mimic the actions we perform in daily life, are the cornerstone of maintaining strength, mobility, and health without the need for a gym. These movements engage multiple muscle groups, improve coordination, and are practical in developing the strength and endurance we need to navigate life's daily challenges.

In this chapter, we'll focus on practical exercises that enhance daily activities such as carrying, lifting, climbing, squatting, and more. By mastering these fundamental movements, you'll not only improve your fitness but also prevent injuries and boost your confidence in handling everyday tasks with ease.

1. The Power of Squats: Strengthen Your Lower Body

Why it's important:

Squatting is one of the most essential functional movements because it replicates actions such as sitting down and standing up, picking up objects from the floor, or getting into and out of a car. Building strong legs and hips through squats helps prevent lower back pain, improves posture, and enhances mobility in everyday life.

How to do it:

- Stand with your feet shoulder-width apart, toes slightly turned out.

- Keep your chest lifted and your back straight as you lower your hips toward the ground, as if you were sitting into an imaginary chair.

- Lower until your thighs are parallel to the floor (or as low as comfortable).

- Push through your heels to stand back up, squeezing your glutes at the top.

Variations:

- Bodyweight Squat: The most basic form, perfect for beginners.

- Goblet Squat: Hold a weight (like a kettlebell or dumbbell) close to your chest to add resistance.

- Single-Leg Squat (Pistol Squat): A more advanced variation that challenges your balance and builds unilateral strength.

Functional Benefit: Squatting enhances your ability to sit down and stand up easily, pick up dropped items without strain, and maintain balance when bending.

2. The Deadlift: Mastering Lifting Techniques

Why it's important:

Lifting objects from the ground is a daily task, whether you're picking up groceries, moving furniture, or loading boxes. The deadlift is the ultimate exercise for teaching proper lifting mechanics and protecting your lower back from injury.

How to do it:

- Stand with your feet hip-width apart, and position the weight (or an imaginary object) in front of your shins.

- Hinge at the hips (not the back) and grip the object with your hands shoulder-width apart.

- Keep your chest up, back straight, and engage your core as you lift by pushing through your heels and straightening your legs and back at the same time.

- Lower the object back to the ground by pushing your hips back, maintaining a flat back throughout the movement.

Variations:

- Kettlebell Deadlift: Using a kettlebell for added weight.

- Single-Leg Deadlift: A great way to work your balance and unilateral leg strength.

Functional Benefit: The deadlift is the key to performing any task that requires bending and lifting, such as picking up boxes, bags, or children without straining your back.

3. The Lunge: Enhancing Mobility and Stability

Why it's important:

Lunges are an excellent functional movement because they mimic the action of stepping forward or climbing stairs. Whether you're carrying groceries up the steps, walking on uneven terrain, or just getting in and out of a car, lunges improve both mobility and stability.

How to do it:

- Stand tall with your feet hip-width apart.

- Step one leg forward, lowering your back knee toward the ground while keeping the front knee over the ankle.

- Push through the heel of the front foot to return to the starting position.

- Alternate legs or complete the reps on one side before switching.

Variations:

- Walking Lunges: Step forward into a lunge, then bring the back foot forward to meet the front foot, and step with the other leg.

- Reverse Lunges: Step backward into the lunge, which is gentler on the knees and helps with balance.

Functional Benefit: Lunges train your body to step and balance, which is essential for walking, climbing stairs, or reacting to changes in terrain.

4. The Push-Up: Building Upper Body Strength for Daily Tasks

Why it's important:

Push-ups engage the chest, shoulders, arms, and core, making them one of the best upper-body exercises for functional fitness. They replicate pushing movements like pushing a door open, lifting a heavy box, or supporting yourself when leaning forward.

How to do it:

- Start in a plank position with your hands slightly wider than shoulder-width apart.

- Keep your body in a straight line from head to heels, with your core engaged.

- Lower your body until your chest almost touches the floor, then push back up to the starting position.

Variations:

- Knee Push-Ups: A modified version for beginners.

- Incline Push-Ups: Place your hands on a raised surface (like a bench) to reduce the difficulty.

- Decline Push-Ups: Elevate your feet to target the upper chest and shoulders more intensely.

Functional Benefit: Push-ups build the strength you need to push, lift, or stabilize objects, making them a great exercise for tasks like opening heavy doors or pushing a cart.

5. The Pull-Up: Building Upper Body Pulling Power

Why it's important:

Pull-ups are one of the best exercises for developing upper body pulling strength. They are essential for actions like climbing, pulling yourself up (such as in a pool or on a ladder), or lifting heavy objects toward you.

How to do it:

- Grab a pull-up bar with an overhand grip, hands slightly wider than shoulder-width.

- Hang with your arms fully extended, and engage your shoulders.

- Pull your body upward until your chin surpasses the bar, then lower yourself back down.

Variations:

- Assisted Pull-Ups: Use a resistance band or pull-up assist machine to help lift your body.

- Negative Pull-Ups: Jump up to the top of the pull-up position and slowly lower yourself down.

Functional Benefit: Pull-ups mimic the action of pulling yourself up or lifting objects towards you, which is essential for climbing and many manual labor tasks.

6. The Carry: Strength for Everyday Transport

Why it's important:

Carrying groceries, moving furniture, or lifting a child requires full-body strength and stability. The carry exercise builds endurance and power for these movements.

How to do it:

- Hold a weight (like a dumbbell, kettlebell, or heavy bag) in one hand.

- Stand tall and engage your core as you walk a set distance, keeping your posture straight and shoulders level.

- Repeat with the other hand or use both hands for a double carry.

Variations:

- Farmer's Walk: Hold a weight in each hand and walk for distance or time.

- Overhead Carry: Hold the weight overhead for an extra challenge to the shoulders and core.

Functional Benefit: The carry enhances your ability to lift, carry, and transport objects with ease and stability, whether it's moving a box or carrying groceries.

Conclusion:

Functional movements are the foundation of everyday strength. They improve how we bend, lift, carry, and move through the world. By regularly incorporating these exercises into your fitness routine, you'll not only build muscle but also enhance your ability to handle daily tasks without injury or fatigue. Whether it's squatting down to pick something up, lunging to step forward, or carrying heavy loads, functional fitness is key to a healthy, independent lifestyle. The best part? You don't need a gym to perform these movements—just your body, some space, and the determination to move with purpose.

CHAPTER 11

OUTDOOR FITNESS ADVENTURES

In today's modern world, many of us are confined to indoor environments for work, leisure, and exercise. The result? A disconnection from nature that can negatively affect both our physical and mental health. Yet, nature has always been the most effective and accessible gym—one that requires no membership fee, no monthly dues, and no sterile equipment. Instead, it offers adventure, freedom, and an incredible range of opportunities for fitness. Whether you're hiking through lush forests, running along winding trails, swimming in a cool lake, or cycling across vast landscapes, the outdoors has something for everyone.

In this chapter, we'll explore some of the best outdoor fitness activities—hiking, trail running, swimming, and cycling—and discuss their many benefits for your body and mind. These activities not only promote physical health but also offer therapeutic effects that help reduce stress, improve mental clarity, and boost overall happiness.

1. Hiking: The Original Full-Body Workout

Hiking is one of the most accessible and versatile outdoor activities you can do, whether you live in the mountains or near flatlands. It's a low-impact activity that doesn't require special skills, making it suitable for individuals of all fitness levels. Whether you're trekking on a gentle path or scaling steep hills, hiking provides an excellent cardiovascular workout while engaging multiple muscle groups.

Benefits of Hiking

- Cardiovascular Health: Hiking at a steady pace elevates your heart rate, promoting heart health and stamina. The more challenging the trail, the greater the cardiovascular benefits.

- Strengthens Muscles: Hiking involves walking, but it also requires you to engage muscles in your legs, hips, core, and even your arms (especially when using trekking poles). Steep inclines or uneven terrain activate stabilizer muscles, helping to improve balance and coordination.

- Mental Health: Nature itself is a great healer. Hiking in the great outdoors reduces anxiety, improves mood, and has been shown to combat feelings of depression. The combination of fresh air, natural beauty, and physical exertion works wonders for your mental state.

The beauty of hiking is its flexibility. You can opt for a gentle walk through a local park, or challenge yourself with a multi-day trek in the mountains. Wherever you choose to hike, remember to start slow, wear proper shoes, and bring plenty of water.

2. Trail Running: The High-Energy Alternative

If you enjoy running but want to break free from the monotony of the treadmill or pavement, trail running is the perfect solution. Running through nature offers a much more dynamic and stimulating experience than a stationary gym workout. The varied terrain forces you to engage more muscles and focus on your surroundings, which makes trail running not only an effective workout but a mental escape as well.

Benefits of Trail Running

- Enhanced Endurance: Running on trails, with their unpredictable surfaces—such as rocks, dirt, and mud—requires more effort than running on flat roads. This builds endurance and stamina over time.

- Reduced Impact: Trail running generally places less strain on your joints than running on concrete or asphalt. The soft dirt trails offer a natural cushion, reducing the risk of injury from overuse.

- Full-Body Workout: While running on a treadmill primarily engages your legs, trail running engages your core and upper body as well. Navigating obstacles and changes in elevation forces you to work harder, improving your agility and strength.

- Stress Relief: Running through scenic landscapes, whether it's a forest, along a coastline, or through a mountain range, is proven to lower stress levels and improve mood. Being immersed in nature has a grounding effect, offering a kind of mindfulness that can help clear your mind and enhance mental clarity.

Trail running can be as challenging or as easy as you make it. Beginners should start on easier paths, gradually increasing distance and difficulty as they build strength. And while the trails are naturally beautiful, always be mindful of the terrain to avoid slips or falls.

3. Swimming: The Ultimate Low-Impact Exercise

Whether you're swimming in the ocean, a lake, or a pool, swimming is one of the best low-impact exercises available. The buoyancy of water reduces the risk of injury, making it a safe choice for people with joint issues or those recovering from injury. Swimming works the entire body, strengthening muscles, improving cardiovascular health, and building endurance, all while being gentle on your joints.

Benefits of Swimming

- Full-Body Conditioning: Swimming engages all major muscle groups, including the legs, arms, back, and core. Whether you're doing the breaststroke, freestyle, or backstroke, you're activating both upper and lower body muscles.

- Cardiovascular Fitness: Swimming is an excellent aerobic activity that gets your heart pumping, improving circulation and promoting overall heart health.

- Mental Well-being: Swimming in natural bodies of water like lakes or oceans is particularly beneficial for mental health. The sound of waves, the rhythm of your strokes, and the sense of freedom from the water can help reduce stress and promote relaxation.

- Improved Flexibility: The fluid motion of swimming enhances flexibility, as the range of motion is often greater in the water than when exercising on land.

Swimming also offers a unique sense of tranquility. The water allows you to focus on your breathing and movement, providing a form of moving meditation. Swimming in open water, like the ocean, can be particularly refreshing and rejuvenating.

4. Cycling: Pedal Your Way to Fitness

Cycling is another versatile outdoor activity that caters to all levels of fitness. Whether you're pedaling around your neighborhood, through the countryside, or on a mountain trail, cycling is a fantastic cardiovascular exercise that also strengthens your legs and core. It's a great alternative for those who want to avoid the repetitive pounding of running or the monotony of gym machines.

Benefits of Cycling

- Cardiovascular Health: Like hiking and running, cycling elevates your heart rate and helps improve cardiovascular health. Whether you're going for a leisurely ride or pushing yourself on a challenging route, cycling can provide both aerobic and anaerobic fitness benefits.

- Leg Strength and Endurance: Cycling primarily targets the lower body, particularly the quads, calves, hamstrings, and glutes. Long rides help build muscular endurance, which translates into better performance in other activities.

- Joint Health: Cycling is a low-impact exercise, making it easier on the joints than activities like running. The circular motion of pedaling avoids the high-impact stresses of other workouts.

- Mental Clarity: Cycling outdoors has a soothing effect on the mind. Exploring new routes, taking in beautiful landscapes, and disconnecting from everyday stress can provide a much-needed mental reset. The focus required for cycling also keeps your mind sharp and engaged.

Cycling can be a solo adventure or a social activity when done in groups. It offers the opportunity to explore new areas, enjoy nature, and get a solid workout all at once.

Conclusion: Adventure Awaits

Outdoor fitness offers the perfect combination of physical activity and immersion in nature. Hiking, trail running, swimming, and cycling are not just effective ways to get fit—they also help reconnect you with the world outside the confines of a gym. Whether you're seeking a peaceful escape or an adrenaline rush, there's an outdoor adventure waiting for you. So, lace up your shoes, grab your gear, and step outside—the natural world is your playground, and it's time to reap the countless rewards that come from fitness in the great outdoors.

CHAPTER 12

THE ART OF PLAY

In the hustle and bustle of adulthood, it's easy to forget the simple joys that come with being active in a carefree way. As children, we naturally engaged in play without a second thought about fitness. We ran, jumped, climbed, and explored, all while laughing and making memories. Yet as we grow older, many of us abandon these activities, thinking of them as childish or unproductive. But what if I told you that the very essence of play could unlock a more vibrant, healthier lifestyle? This chapter is about rediscovering the art of play and how embracing these activities can reduce stress, improve fitness, and enhance your well-being in ways traditional workouts often can't.

Rediscovering Play: It's Not Just for Kids

Play is a natural, instinctual form of movement that we all engage in as children. We jump, run, throw, kick, climb, and explore—all of it without any external motivation other than the pure joy of the activity. These simple actions build our physical skills, strengthen our bodies, and stimulate our brains. Yet, as adults, play often becomes relegated to the background of our busy lives.

Many adults mistakenly believe that fitness has to be serious, structured, and goal-oriented. The gym, weightlifting, running on a treadmill—these are seen as the true avenues to a fit and healthy body. While there's no denying the importance of exercise, the rigid, regimented approach can feel draining and uninspiring over time.

The truth is, play is a powerful, underrated form of exercise. It taps into our primal need for movement, brings joy, and fosters creativity, all while providing the benefits of physical exertion. When we engage in playful activities, we're not just burning calories—we're reconnecting with a deeper, more instinctive way of moving our bodies.

The Many Forms of Play

Play takes many forms, and the beauty of it is that it's adaptable to your environment, your interests, and your fitness goals. Here are just a few examples of childhood activities that not only reignite nostalgia but also serve as excellent ways to stay fit:

1. Jumping Rope

Jumping rope is one of the most effective cardiovascular exercises, and it's also a playful and fun way to work out. It enhances coordination, balance, and agility while providing a full-body workout. Whether you're hopping in the backyard or in a park, the rhythmic motion of the rope combined with the joy of jumping like a kid will make it feel more like play than exercise. As you get better, you can incorporate tricks, speed, and endurance challenges to keep it engaging.

2. Playing Tag

Tag is one of those activities that taps directly into your inner child. Running around, dodging and weaving in an unpredictable game of tag, engages your cardiovascular system, builds speed, and improves reflexes. The unpredictable nature of tag keeps you on your toes, demanding full-body coordination and sharp mental focus. You'll be surprised at how quickly your heart rate rises and how much you're sweating, all while laughing and competing with friends or family.

3. Climbing Trees

The childhood pastime of climbing trees does far more than just bring a sense of adventure. It strengthens the muscles in your arms, legs, and core while improving flexibility, balance, and coordination. It's also a great way to reconnect with nature. The freedom of climbing offers an intense physical workout that requires strength, control, and agility—skills that are often overlooked in conventional exercise routines.

4. Hula Hooping

Hula hooping may seem like a fun activity from the past, but it's an excellent way to work your core. Twisting and turning to keep the hoop in motion engages your abdominal muscles, improving your posture and stability. It's a simple, fun movement that can be done anywhere, and there's no pressure to be perfect. You simply flow with the hoop, losing yourself in the rhythm of it.

5. Dance Parties

Who says you need to be in a club or a class to dance? Put on your favorite music and have a spontaneous dance party in your living room, on your balcony, or in your backyard. Dancing is an excellent cardiovascular workout, and the joy it brings can significantly improve your mood. Whether you're doing an impromptu solo routine or dancing with friends, it's a playful and effective way to boost both your fitness and mental health.

How Play Reduces Stress and Improves Fitness

Playful activities not only make fitness feel less like a chore, but they also have a remarkable ability to reduce stress. Life can be overwhelming—work, family obligations, and personal responsibilities pile up, leaving little room for relaxation or fun. When we engage in playful, carefree activities, we temporarily shift our focus away from those stresses. Here's how play helps:

1. Stress Reduction

Play releases endorphins, the body's natural "feel-good" chemicals. These endorphins reduce feelings of anxiety and stress, enhancing our mood and sense of well-being. Engaging in fun activities like jumping rope or playing tag can serve as a natural stress reliever, allowing you to disconnect from the pressures of everyday life. The laughter and lightheartedness that come with play are some of the most potent antidotes to stress.

2. Improved Mental Health

Physical activity through play also promotes mental clarity and emotional resilience. When we engage in an activity that doesn't feel like "exercise," we're often able to let go of mental tension, gaining a new perspective on problems and challenges. Play encourages mindfulness—being fully present in the moment, whether you're jumping in a puddle or sprinting away from someone in a game of tag.

3. Increased Motivation

One of the barriers many adults face with traditional exercise is the sense of obligation. "I have to work out," they think. But when you make fitness feel like play, it becomes something you want to do. Because play is intrinsically enjoyable, you're more likely to stick with it, which leads to improved fitness outcomes over time. It encourages regular movement, which is the key to long-term health.

4. Physical Fitness Gains

While play is fun, it's also highly effective. Jumping rope can improve cardiovascular fitness and leg strength. Running around in a game of tag builds speed and endurance. Climbing trees increases upper body strength. Even something as simple as chasing a ball or jumping over hurdles can enhance coordination, balance, and flexibility.

5. Social Connection

Play often involves others, and this social element is crucial for both mental and physical well-being. Whether you're playing tag with kids, dancing with friends, or challenging a sibling to a jump rope contest, these moments of shared joy help to strengthen bonds, reduce feelings of isolation, and foster a sense of community.

Bringing Play Into Your Life

Now that you understand the benefits of play, the next step is incorporating it into your life. Start small—take a few minutes each day to engage in a playful activity. Maybe it's a quick game of tag with your kids, a solo hula hooping session in the backyard, or even a dance party in your living room. The goal isn't to force yourself to work out but to embrace play as a natural part of your routine.

You don't need a fancy gym or equipment. All you need is the willingness to let go of any judgment and rediscover the joy of movement. Let play remind you that fitness can—and should—be fun.

CHAPTER 13

LOW-IMPACT FITNESS FOR LONGEVITY

In the pursuit of fitness, many people gravitate toward high-intensity workouts to achieve quick results. However, these intense regimens often neglect an important aspect of fitness—longevity. As we age, our bodies require a fitness approach that prioritizes joint health, flexibility, and recovery to ensure we remain active and pain-free for as long as possible. Low-impact fitness is not only gentle on the body but also incredibly effective for improving mobility, strength, and overall wellness.

In this chapter, we'll explore the benefits of yoga, Pilates, and stretching routines as tools to protect your joints, enhance recovery, and promote long-term health.

The Power of Yoga

Yoga is one of the most effective low-impact activities available. It's a holistic practice that nurtures the body, mind, and spirit, focusing on flexibility, strength, and breath control. While yoga may appear slow or gentle compared to high-impact exercises, it offers a range of benefits that contribute to lifelong fitness.

1. Improving Flexibility and Mobility

Flexibility is crucial for joint health, particularly as we age. Regular yoga practice can help lengthen muscles, release tension, and increase range of motion. By improving flexibility, yoga reduces stiffness in the joints, alleviating discomfort and enhancing mobility. For those with chronic pain, conditions like arthritis, or stiffness in specific areas (such as the lower back or hips), yoga can serve as a restorative practice to loosen tight muscles and improve movement.

Common yoga poses like the Downward Dog, Child's Pose, and Cat-Cow stretches the spine and lower back, while Pigeon Pose and Hip Openers target the hips and legs. Through controlled breathing and deliberate movement, yoga ensures that these stretches are done gently, without overstretching, which can lead to injury.

2. Building Strength and Stability

While yoga is often associated with flexibility, it is also a powerful strength-building tool. Many yoga poses require you to hold your body in specific positions, which engages deep stabilizing muscles. Plank Pose, Warrior Poses, and Chair Pose strengthen the core, legs, arms, and back, helping to create a strong foundation that supports your joints.

This combination of strength and flexibility is essential for injury prevention and longevity. Strong muscles help protect the joints by supporting them more effectively, reducing the risk of wear and tear, and alleviating strain during everyday activities.

3. Stress Relief and Mental Health

Yoga's focus on mindfulness, breathing, and meditation also promotes mental well-being. Chronic stress can exacerbate physical issues like muscle tightness, joint pain, and poor posture. Yoga offers a calming and centering practice that helps reduce stress hormones and improve mood, making it an essential part of overall health and longevity.

Pilates: Strength Through Control

Pilates is another low-impact exercise system that focuses on controlled movements, core strength, and improving posture. Created by Joseph Pilates in the early 20th century, Pilates combines strength training with flexibility exercises to create a balanced body. While similar to yoga, Pilates emphasizes core engagement and focuses more on precise movement and alignment.

1. Strengthening the Core

A strong core is the foundation of all movement. Pilates is renowned for its ability to engage and strengthen the deep abdominal muscles, which are vital for maintaining a healthy spine and preventing back pain. The exercises in Pilates teach you to control your muscles, making them more functional in everyday life.

Core strength is essential for maintaining good posture, reducing the risk of falls, and protecting the lower back from injury. By improving the strength of the transversus abdominis (the deepest layer of abdominal muscles), Pilates helps to stabilize the spine and pelvis, ensuring efficient movement patterns.

2. Enhancing Posture and Alignment

Many people experience poor posture due to prolonged sitting, sedentary lifestyles, or improper movement patterns. Over time, poor posture can lead to muscle imbalances, pain, and even joint degeneration. Pilates, with its focus on proper alignment and posture, teaches you to engage the correct muscles, which improves your overall body alignment.

Through exercises like The Roll Up, The Saw, and Spine Stretch, Pilates helps to elongate the spine and realign the body. Improved posture not only reduces strain on the muscles and joints but also increases energy levels and promotes better digestion.

3. Rehabilitation and Injury Prevention

Pilates is often used in rehabilitation settings because of its low-impact, gentle approach to building strength and mobility. It's ideal for people recovering from injury or surgery, as it focuses on controlled movements that prevent strain and encourage proper healing. The practice also works to correct muscle imbalances and improve flexibility, which can prevent future injuries.

Stretching: The Foundation of Flexibility and Joint Protection

Stretching is often overlooked in fitness routines, yet it's a crucial element of a low-impact workout regimen. Stretching improves flexibility, reduces muscle tension, enhances circulation, and promotes joint health. A well-rounded stretching routine can be done daily to maintain mobility and reduce the risk of injury.

1. Dynamic Stretching: Preparing the Body for Movement

Before any workout, it's important to prepare your body with dynamic stretching—active stretches that move through a full range of motion. Dynamic stretching helps increase blood flow to the muscles, improving flexibility and reducing the likelihood of strains or pulls. Examples include leg swings, arm circles, and walking lunges.

Dynamic stretches are particularly beneficial before engaging in cardio or resistance training, as they warm up the muscles and prepare them for movement.

2. Static Stretching: Enhancing Flexibility and Recovery

After exercise, static stretching involves holding a stretch for 20–30 seconds to lengthen the muscles and relax them. Static stretches help improve overall flexibility and counteract the tightness that can accumulate in muscles during activity. Common stretches like the hamstring stretch, quad stretch, and shoulder stretch allow the body to return to a relaxed state, aiding in muscle recovery.

Focusing on stretching major muscle groups like the hamstrings, calves, back, and shoulders can relieve post-workout soreness and tightness, enhancing recovery and reducing the risk of stiffness.

3. The Importance of Joint Mobility

Joints benefit significantly from stretching, as it improves synovial fluid production and increases joint range of motion. Stretching helps reduce the wear and tear on joints, particularly in areas like the knees, hips, and shoulders. Incorporating joint mobility exercises, such as gentle hip circles, wrist stretches, and ankle rotations, can prevent stiffness and keep your joints flexible.

Conclusion: The Longevity of Low-Impact Fitness

The beauty of low-impact fitness lies in its accessibility, safety, and effectiveness. Yoga, Pilates, and stretching are not only gentle on the body, but they also nurture it, promoting mobility, strength, and overall wellness. By incorporating these practices into your daily life, you can protect your joints, recover effectively from physical activity, and enhance your overall longevity. Whether you are a beginner or someone with years of experience, these exercises offer lifelong benefits to keep your body moving well into your later years.

Incorporating yoga, Pilates, and stretching routines into your fitness regimen will help you stay agile, flexible, and strong. With consistency and mindfulness, you'll create a foundation for health that endures.

CHAPTER 14

UILDING STRENGTH WITH MINIMAL EQUIPMENT

When it comes to building strength, the idea that you need a fully equipped gym is one of the most misleading myths in fitness. While commercial gyms boast rows of heavy weights and machines, the truth is that your body and a few simple tools are all you need to achieve significant strength gains. Resistance bands, pull-up bars, and even household items can be used to create an effective and efficient workout routine. This chapter will show you how to harness the power of minimal equipment to build strength, save money, and maintain a workout routine that fits into your life—without ever stepping foot in a gym.

The Power of Resistance Bands

Resistance bands are one of the most versatile and affordable pieces of equipment you can incorporate into your routine. They're small, lightweight, and can be used to work virtually every muscle in the body, making them perfect for strength training at home or on the go.

Why Resistance Bands Work

The beauty of resistance bands lies in the constant tension they create throughout the movement, which forces your muscles to work harder. Unlike free weights, which you only lift during the upward phase, resistance bands apply tension through both the concentric (shortening) and eccentric (lengthening) phases of movement. This means that you're engaging your muscles more thoroughly, improving strength and muscle tone.

Key Resistance Band Exercises

1. Squats: Stand with your feet shoulder-width apart, holding the resistance band under your feet with both hands at shoulder height. Squat down, pushing your hips back, and rise up against the tension of the band. This works your quads, glutes, and core.

2. Chest Press: Anchor the band behind you (like the door or a sturdy post). Hold the handles, step forward, and press the bands forward, elbows bent at 90 degrees. This targets the chest and shoulders.

3. Rows: Sit on the floor with your legs extended in front of you, wrapping the resistance band around your feet. Pull the handles towards you, squeezing your shoulder blades together. Rows work the back muscles and biceps.

4. Lateral Band Walks: Place a resistance band around your legs just above the knees. Stand with feet shoulder-width apart and squat slightly. Step to the side, maintaining tension on the band. This works the hip abductors and glutes.

Resistance bands come in different resistance levels, from light to heavy. You can easily adjust the intensity by shortening the length of the band or adding more resistance. This allows for progression as you get stronger.

Mastering Pull-Ups at Home

Pull-ups are one of the best exercises for building upper body strength, particularly targeting the back, shoulders, and arms. However, the ability to do a pull-up is something that many people struggle with initially. The good news is that you don't need a gym to do them—just a pull-up bar and a little practice.

Why Pull-Ups Matter

Pull-ups engage multiple muscle groups, including the lats, biceps, and forearms. They are considered a compound movement, meaning they require the coordination of various muscles and joints. This makes them an excellent functional exercise for overall strength and upper body development.

Installing a Pull-Up Bar

Many inexpensive and space-saving pull-up bars are designed to fit in doorframes, so you don't need a special gym setup to add this tool to your fitness routine. Choose a sturdy bar that can safely hold your weight.

Assisted Pull-Ups

If you can't do a full pull-up yet, resistance bands can help. Simply attach the band to the pull-up bar, loop it around your knees or feet, and it will assist you as you pull yourself up. This allows you to build strength gradually.

Pull-Up Progression

1. Negative Pull-Ups: Start with your chin over the bar (you can use a stool or jump to get there). Slowly lower yourself down, resisting gravity for as long as possible. Negative reps help build the strength necessary for a full pull-up.

2. Scapular Pull-Ups: Hang from the bar with your arms fully extended. Without bending your elbows, squeeze your shoulder blades down and back. This helps to activate the muscles required for a proper pull-up.

3. Inverted Rows: If you're not yet able to do pull-ups, inverted rows are a great alternative. Set a bar (or use a sturdy table) at waist height. Lie underneath, grasp the bar, and pull your chest up toward it.

By using a pull-up bar and incorporating assisted pull-ups or progressions, you can eventually build the strength needed to perform full pull-ups without additional equipment.

Using Household Items for Strength Training

One of the easiest ways to build strength without spending a dime is to look around your home. Everyday objects can become useful tools for your strength training workout. By simply being resourceful, you can avoid the high costs of fancy fitness tools.

Common Household Items and Their Uses:

1. Backpack with Books (or Other Weights):

   - Fill a backpack with books or water bottles for added resistance. You can use it for squats, lunges, or even weighted push-ups.

   - Squats with a Backpack: Place the backpack on your shoulders, squat down, and stand back up. The added weight challenges your lower body.

2. Chairs and Tables for Dips and Elevated Push-Ups:

- Use a sturdy chair or table to perform tricep dips. Place your hands behind you on the chair, legs extended, and lower your body down.

- Elevated Push-Ups: Use a low table or chair to elevate your feet during push-ups. This increases the intensity and shifts the focus to your upper chest and shoulders.

3. Water Bottles or Cans as Dumbbells:

- Use full water bottles, soup cans, or any small household item as makeshift dumbbells for bicep curls, overhead presses, or lateral raises.

- Bicep Curls: Hold a water bottle in each hand, keeping your elbows stationary, and curl the bottles towards your shoulders.

4. Towels for Resistance:

- Towels can be used to perform towel rows. Loop a towel around a door handle and pull it toward your body, engaging your back muscles.

- Towel Rows: With your feet planted, grab the towel with both hands and lean back, then pull yourself toward the door.

5. Ladders and Steps for Step-Ups:

   - Use the first step of your staircase for step-ups. Alternate legs as you step up, engaging your quads and glutes.

   - Lunges with a Step-Up: Add a lunge after each step-up to increase difficulty and work the lower body.

DIY Alternatives to Expensive Fitness Tools

If you prefer to use specialized equipment, consider DIY alternatives that mimic their function but are far more cost-effective.

1. Sandbags: Instead of buying expensive weight bags, fill a sturdy duffel bag with sand or gravel to create your own adjustable sandbag. Sandbags are excellent for squats, lunges, and overhead presses, and they provide an unstable surface, which challenges your core stability.

2. Homemade Medicine Ball: Use a basketball or soccer ball and fill it with sand, dirt, or rice to create a medicine ball. Medicine ball exercises like slams and tosses are great for building explosive power.

3. PVC Pipe Resistance Bar: You can make your own resistance bar by attaching resistance bands to a PVC pipe. This allows for barbell-like movements such as squats and deadlifts without the heavy weight.

Conclusion

Building strength without a gym doesn't require complicated equipment or expensive tools. With resistance bands, a pull-up bar, household items, and a little creativity, you can achieve incredible results at home or anywhere. The key is consistency, progressive overload, and using the tools that work best for you. By incorporating minimal equipment into your workout routine, you'll not only save time and money but also develop functional strength that improves your day-to-day life.

Remember: your body is the most powerful tool you have. have. Equip it with the right resources and let it do the work.

CHAPTER 15

THE ROLE OF MARTIAL ARTS AND DANCE

When we think of fitness, the first images that often come to mind are weights, treadmills, or maybe yoga mats. However, fitness isn't confined to traditional exercises. Some of the most effective and holistic workouts come from ancient practices and creative expression, where movement is the key to physical and mental wellness. Martial arts and dance not only offer a great way to get fit, but they also provide the mind-body connection that many conventional gym routines lack. From the graceful flow of tai chi to the high-energy strikes of kickboxing and the rhythmic sway of salsa, these movement-focused disciplines offer a full-body workout like no other.

Tai Chi: The Art of Mindful Movement

Tai chi, often referred to as "meditation in motion," is a gentle martial art originating from China. It is known for its slow, controlled movements, deep breathing, and mindfulness. Despite its calm and fluid nature, tai chi is a powerful workout that enhances balance, flexibility, and strength.

One of the primary benefits of tai chi is its emphasis on control and body awareness. As practitioners move through sequences of postures, they focus on aligning their body and mind, working to achieve fluidity in movement. This meditative quality makes tai chi particularly effective for reducing stress while improving coordination. The slow tempo allows beginners to master each movement with precision, making it accessible to people of all fitness levels, including older adults or those recovering from injury.

From a physical perspective, tai chi builds strength and balance through its weight-shifting movements. By standing on one leg, transitioning weight from foot to foot, and holding poses for extended periods, practitioners engage muscles throughout the entire body. The slow movements force muscles to maintain tension for longer, offering a muscular endurance workout. Additionally, tai chi has been shown to enhance flexibility and joint mobility, which can help reduce the risk of falls and promote overall body awareness.

In terms of cardiovascular benefits, tai chi may not be as intense as high-intensity training, but research has shown it can improve heart health by lowering blood pressure and promoting circulation. The deep breathing exercises also stimulate the parasympathetic nervous system, encouraging relaxation and reducing the physical effects of stress.

Tai chi's true strength lies in its ability to unite the body and mind. The practice encourages a flow of energy (often referred to as "Qi") throughout the body, increasing mental clarity and emotional balance. The meditation aspect of tai chi brings mental calmness, improving focus and reducing anxiety, making it not only an excellent physical workout but also a tool for emotional health.

Kickboxing: A Full-Body Workout

Kickboxing is a dynamic, high-intensity martial art that combines elements of traditional boxing with powerful kicks. Known for its speed and explosive movements, kickboxing offers a total-body workout that improves cardiovascular endurance, muscular strength, and coordination.

What makes kickboxing an outstanding workout is its full-body engagement. Every punch, kick, and knee strike targets multiple muscle groups simultaneously. The arms work in tandem with the core and legs, creating a high-calorie burn that boosts metabolism. Kicking exercises strengthen the quads, hamstrings, and glutes, while punches work the shoulders, biceps, and chest. Core muscles are heavily involved in stabilizing the body during both punches and kicks, making kickboxing an excellent way to develop a strong midsection.

Kickboxing is an incredible cardiovascular workout. The combination of high-energy rounds and short recovery intervals leads to an increase in heart rate and improved stamina. The aerobic benefits of kickboxing help build endurance while also burning fat, making it an ideal workout for those looking to lose weight or improve overall fitness.

Additionally, kickboxing is a fantastic stress reliever. The intensity of the workout and the focus required to throw punches and kicks can provide a cathartic release of built-up tension and frustration. The mental concentration needed to master the various techniques also increases mental toughness and discipline. As with most martial arts, kickboxing can also boost confidence as practitioners see improvements in both their physical abilities and mental resilience.

Kickboxing classes often include shadowboxing, bag work, and sparring, all of which improve reaction time and coordination. The athleticism and speed required to perform quick, powerful movements make kickboxing a dynamic workout for people seeking a high-intensity, results-driven routine.

Salsa Dancing: Fun and Fitness Combined

If kickboxing offers intensity and tai chi brings mindfulness, salsa dancing combines fun with fitness. Salsa, a Latin dance style with roots in Afro-Cuban and Puerto Rican culture, is a rhythmic dance that involves fast footwork, hip movements, and partner coordination. What sets salsa apart from other fitness activities is the joy and excitement it brings while still providing a heart-pumping workout.

Salsa dancing is an excellent cardiovascular exercise. The fast-paced footwork and continuous movement keep your heart rate elevated, providing an aerobic workout that can improve heart health, increase endurance, and burn calories. Unlike a treadmill workout, salsa dancing is more engaging, making it easy to forget you're even exercising.

One of the most appealing aspects of salsa is its ability to work the whole body. The movement involves fluid hip rotations, legwork, and upper-body engagement, which strengthens the core and improves flexibility. The dance's emphasis on rhythmic movement enhances coordination, balance, and agility. The constant shifting of weight between the feet and swift turns also builds lower body strength and stability.

Moreover, salsa dancing is a social activity, and the connection with others brings a mental health benefit that traditional workouts lack. Social engagement has been linked to a reduction in feelings of isolation and depression, making salsa dancing not just a way to stay fit but also a way to connect with others and improve your mood.

Salsa is also an excellent way to develop timing and rhythm. These skills transfer to other areas of life and fitness, helping improve your coordination in both dance and daily activities. As with other dance styles, salsa provides an avenue for creativity and self-expression. It allows people to move freely to the music, which can be both liberating and empowering.

Why Martial Arts and Dance Are So Effective

Whether it's the mindfulness of tai chi, the intensity of kickboxing, or the rhythm of salsa dancing, martial arts and dance offer a uniquely holistic approach to fitness. These movement-based disciplines combine cardiovascular, strength, and flexibility training, all while engaging the mind in ways that many traditional workouts cannot.

The appeal of martial arts and dance lies in their versatility. They can be adapted for different fitness levels, can be done solo or in groups, and are often accessible with minimal equipment. Most importantly, they make fitness fun. When you're having fun, you're more likely to stick with the activity, making it easier to integrate these practices into your daily life.

Incorporating martial arts or dance into your fitness routine not only helps you get fit but also teaches you valuable skills such as discipline, coordination, and confidence. Whether you're seeking strength, endurance, flexibility, or mental clarity, these movement-focused disciplines offer the full-body workout that will transform both your body and your mind.

CHAPTER 16

NUTRITION AS FUEL

Fitness isn't just about lifting weights, running, or doing bodyweight exercises; it's also about how you fuel your body. Nutrition is an essential piece of the puzzle that ensures you perform at your best and recover effectively. But the goal isn't to get bogged down by calorie counting or restrictive diets. Instead, the key lies in understanding and balancing your macronutrients—proteins, carbohydrates, and fats—and knowing how they impact your body's energy levels, performance, and recovery.

Balancing Macronutrients

Macronutrients are the building blocks of your diet and include protein, carbohydrates, and fats. Each of these macronutrients plays a specific role in supporting your body's needs, particularly when you're engaging in regular exercise. By understanding the purpose of each and how to balance them throughout the day, you can fuel your body without obsessing over calories.

Protein: Building and Repairing Muscle

Protein is often the most talked about macronutrient in fitness circles, and for good reason. It is the primary building block of muscle tissue, and after a workout, your muscles need protein to repair and grow. Consuming enough protein helps support recovery, maintain lean muscle mass, and improve overall strength.

But how much protein do you need? The general guideline for active individuals is to aim for about 0.8 to 1 gram of protein per pound of body weight. This might sound like a lot, but it's often easier to meet this target than most people think. Protein-rich foods include chicken, turkey, fish, tofu, lentils, beans, eggs, and dairy products.

Carbohydrates: The Body's Primary Energy Source

Carbohydrates often get a bad reputation, but they are the body's primary source of energy, particularly during intense exercise. When you consume carbohydrates, they are broken down into glucose, which your muscles use for energy. Without sufficient carbohydrates, you may feel sluggish, have trouble sustaining energy during a workout, or recover poorly afterward.

There are two types of carbohydrates: simple and complex. Simple carbs (like sugar and white bread) provide quick energy but can lead to spikes and crashes in blood sugar. On the other hand, complex carbs (such as whole grains, sweet potatoes, and fruits) provide sustained energy and are loaded with fiber, which is good for digestion and overall health.

Depending on your exercise intensity and goals, carbohydrates should make up around 40-60% of your total daily intake. A higher carbohydrate intake is especially important if you are engaging in high-intensity workouts, long endurance activities, or trying to gain muscle mass.

Fats: The Unsung Heroes of Energy and Health

Fats are essential for a variety of bodily functions, from hormone production to protecting your organs. Fats are also important for keeping you satisfied after meals, which helps prevent overeating. They are slower to digest than carbs, providing long-lasting energy.

Healthy fats, such as those found in avocados, olive oil, nuts, seeds, and fatty fish (like salmon), should be prioritized over unhealthy fats, which can be found in processed foods, fried foods, and trans fats. Aim to incorporate fats into every meal for balanced energy throughout the day.

Fats should make up about 20-30% of your daily intake, depending on your goals. If you're aiming for muscle gain, you might need a bit more, but for general fitness and health, focusing on healthy fats in moderation is key.

Pre-Workout Nutrition: Energizing Your Body for Performance

What you eat before a workout can have a significant impact on your performance. Your goal with pre-workout nutrition is to fuel your body with the right amount of energy, ensuring you have enough glycogen in your muscles to perform your best.

Timing and Composition:

- Aim to eat a balanced meal about 1 to 2 hours before your workout. This allows enough time for digestion and energy absorption.

- Focus on a combination of complex carbohydrates (for sustained energy) and protein (for muscle repair). Keep the fat content relatively low before exercise, as fats take longer to digest.

Pre-Workout Meal Ideas:

- Oatmeal with almond butter and berries: A great source of complex carbs, healthy fats, and a touch of protein.

- Greek yogurt with honey and granola: Packed with protein and carbs to fuel your muscles.

- Whole grain toast with avocado and a boiled egg: A satisfying, balanced option for slow-releasing energy.

- Smoothie with banana, spinach, protein powder, and almond milk: Easy to digest, hydrating, and energizing.

These options provide a good balance of macronutrients that will help you perform well during your workout.

Post-Workout Nutrition: Maximizing Recovery

After your workout, your body is in a prime state to recover and repair muscle tissue. Post-workout nutrition is critical for replenishing glycogen stores, repairing muscle fibers, and reducing inflammation. The key is to consume a meal or snack that includes protein, carbs, and some healthy fats.

Timing and Composition:

- Ideally, you want to consume your post-workout meal within 30 to 60 minutes after finishing your workout. This is when your body's nutrient absorption is at its peak.

- Focus on high-quality protein for muscle repair and carbohydrates to replenish glycogen stores. A small amount of fat can also help promote long-term recovery but shouldn't be the focus immediately post-workout.

Post-Workout Meal Ideas:

- Grilled chicken with quinoa and steamed vegetables: A perfect balance of protein and carbs, with fiber for digestion.

- Protein shake with banana and almond butter: Quick, convenient, and protein-packed to support muscle recovery.

- Tuna salad with mixed greens and olive oil: A protein-packed meal with healthy fats to support recovery.

- Sweet potato with cottage cheese and a handful of nuts: A great option to replenish glycogen stores and repair muscles.

These meals will not only aid in muscle recovery but also keep your energy levels stable post-workout.

Final Thoughts: Food as Fuel, Not Foe

Remember that fueling your body doesn't have to be a meticulous, calorie-counting process. Instead, focus on balanced meals that nourish your body and support your fitness goals. By incorporating sufficient amounts of protein, carbohydrates, and healthy fats into your diet, you'll have the energy to crush your workouts and the nutrients to recover effectively. Prioritize whole, nutrient-dense foods, and avoid the extremes of fad diets or restrictive eating. Fitness is about feeling strong, healthy, and energized—and that begins with proper nutrition.

With the right balance of macronutrients, your body will thank you by performing at its best, both in and out of the gym (or, in your case, in your home or outdoors).

CHAPTER 17

RECOVERY: THE HIDDEN KEY TO PROGRESS

In the pursuit of fitness, we often focus on the "doing" part: the workouts, the running, the weightlifting, and the sweat. But here's the truth—none of it matters if you don't allow your body the time it needs to rest, recover, and rebuild. Recovery is often the most overlooked aspect of fitness, yet it plays an indispensable role in progress. Without proper recovery, all the hard work you put in could be in vain. This chapter will explore the importance of recovery, the key elements involved, and how to incorporate them into your fitness routine to ensure sustainable growth.

The Role of Sleep in Recovery

If you've ever felt sluggish after a night of poor sleep or found your performance dipping despite training hard, it's no coincidence. Sleep is your body's ultimate recovery tool. When we sleep, the body is not only resting, but also engaging in critical processes that repair muscles, replenish energy stores, and regulate hormones. This is when muscle growth happens—during deep sleep, growth hormone production spikes, aiding in tissue repair and protein synthesis.

Lack of sleep or poor-quality sleep inhibits these processes, leading to longer recovery times, reduced performance, and a higher risk of injury. In fact, studies have shown that sleep deprivation can negatively affect strength, endurance, and cognitive function. Whether you're doing bodyweight exercises or endurance training, sleep is the most powerful ally you have.

How much sleep do you need? While individual needs vary, most adults require between 7-9 hours of quality sleep per night. To optimize recovery, aim for consistent sleep patterns by going to bed and waking up at the same time each day. Create a sleep-friendly environment: keep your room dark, quiet, and cool, and avoid screens for at least an hour before bed to allow your body to produce the necessary melatonin for rest.

Rest Days: The Secret to Progress

Many fitness enthusiasts make the mistake of pushing their bodies too hard, believing that more is always better. However, rest days are a fundamental part of any effective fitness program. These are the days when the body gets the opportunity to repair and strengthen itself after intense workouts. If you don't allow for adequate rest, your muscles won't have time to rebuild, and you might even experience the dreaded burnout or overtraining syndrome.

Rest days can vary in intensity. It's important to note that rest doesn't necessarily mean complete inactivity—it could also mean doing something low-impact that promotes circulation and flexibility. On your rest days, you could take a light walk, do some gentle yoga, or engage in other forms of movement that don't stress your muscles excessively. This kind of active recovery helps maintain mobility and reduces soreness without overtaxing the body.

The general rule of thumb is to take one to two full rest days per week, depending on your training intensity and goals. If you're doing high-intensity training (HIIT, heavy lifting, etc.), you may need more rest days. Listen to your body—it will tell you when it's time to ease off. Persistent soreness, fatigue, or a plateau in performance are signs you may need to scale back and focus on recovery.

Active Recovery: Resting with Purpose

Active recovery is a technique that involves engaging in low-intensity activities on rest days, which helps your body recover while staying active. The goal is to keep blood flowing to muscles, which promotes the healing of micro-tears in the muscle fibers caused by intense exercise. While full rest days are important, active recovery can speed up the healing process and reduce soreness.

Some great active recovery activities include:

- Walking or light jogging: These activities are excellent for improving circulation without placing stress on your body.

- Swimming: A low-impact exercise that allows your body to move through water, providing resistance while being easy on the joints.

- Yoga and stretching: These help improve flexibility and decrease muscle tightness, making it easier for muscles to recover and function optimally.

- Cycling: A low-impact form of cardio that helps improve endurance while allowing the muscles to recover from more intense workouts.

Incorporating these gentle activities into your routine will promote mobility, reduce stiffness, and enhance recovery while still allowing you to move.

Tools for Recovery: Foam Rollers, Stretching, and Massages

While sleep, rest days, and active recovery are essential, there are additional tools and techniques you can use to speed up recovery and keep your body in peak condition.

1. Foam Rolling:

Foam rolling is a form of self-myofascial release (SMR), a technique that targets tight muscles and fascia (the connective tissue around muscles). When you foam roll, you apply pressure to different areas of your body, helping to release knots, increase blood flow, and improve flexibility. By regularly using a foam roller, you can reduce muscle soreness, enhance mobility, and prevent the buildup of scar tissue.

How to foam roll:

Focus on the major muscle groups—quads, hamstrings, calves, back, and glutes. Roll each area slowly for about 30 seconds to 1 minute, applying gentle pressure. If you hit a tender spot, pause and allow the muscle to release. Avoid rolling directly over joints or bones.

2. Stretching:

Stretching is one of the simplest and most effective ways to prevent tightness and promote recovery. After a workout, your muscles are often shortened and tight, and stretching helps to lengthen them, improving flexibility and reducing stiffness. Incorporating dynamic stretches (leg swings, arm circles) before your workout and static stretches (holding a stretch for 20-30 seconds) afterward will help maintain your range of motion and prevent injury.

Key areas to focus on include your hamstrings, hip flexors, quads, shoulders, and back. These are common trouble spots for tightness, especially if you're working at a desk or spending long hours in a seated position.

3. Massages:

While professional massages can be expensive, using a massage gun or even performing self-massage with your hands can have similar benefits. Massage helps to alleviate muscle tension, improve circulation, and promote relaxation. Whether you use a massage ball to target your back or a handheld massage gun to focus on specific muscles, these tools can help reduce soreness and speed up recovery.

For targeted relief, try massaging tight areas for 5-10 minutes, using circular motions and applying enough pressure to release tension without causing discomfort.

Conclusion

Recovery is not an afterthought—it is a vital component of any successful fitness regimen. Without sufficient sleep, rest days, and proper recovery tools, your progress will plateau, and you risk injury. By incorporating these recovery strategies into your routine, you ensure that your body has the time and support it needs to grow stronger, more resilient, and prepared for the next challenge. Remember, in fitness, less can often be more. Allow your body to rest, recharge, and rebuild—and you'll see the results not only in the gym but in every aspect of your life.

CHAPTER 18

TRACKING PROGRESS WITHOUT OVERWHELM

When embarking on a fitness journey without the confines of a gym, one of the challenges you might face is tracking your progress. Without scales or machines to measure your improvements, it's easy to become uncertain of whether you're on the right path. However, tracking doesn't have to be a source of stress or overwhelm. It can become an enjoyable and empowering part of your routine, helping you stay focused, motivated, and connected to your goals.

In this chapter, we'll explore practical methods to measure your progress—through stamina, strength, and flexibility—along with simple tools like journaling, habit tracking, and wearable technology to support your journey.

Measuring Progress Through Stamina

Stamina is the capacity to sustain physical activity over an extended period, whether it's running, cycling, or simply being active for longer periods without feeling exhausted. Tracking your stamina allows you to gauge how well your body adapts to increasing demands and improving endurance. Unlike strength or flexibility, stamina is often most easily measured by how long or how intensely you can perform a specific activity.

To track stamina without getting overwhelmed, use the following approaches:

1. Distance and Time:

Start by tracking the duration of your workouts or the distance you cover. For example, if you're a runner or a cyclist, you can monitor how long it takes to complete a certain distance or how far you can go in a set amount of time. If you run or cycle in your neighborhood, set a baseline time and distance for your first attempt. In subsequent weeks, aim to reduce the time it takes or increase the distance.

2. Heart Rate Monitoring:

Your heart rate is a great indicator of your cardiovascular endurance. Using a simple wristwatch or a fitness band with heart rate monitoring can help you track how hard your heart is working during exercise. Over time, as your stamina improves, you'll notice that it takes a lower heart rate to complete the same activity, which indicates increased cardiovascular health.

3. Perceived Effort:

The Rating of Perceived Exertion (RPE) scale can help you track how challenging an activity feels. On a scale from 1 to 10 (where 1 is very easy and 10 is extremely difficult), record how hard a workout feels at the end. As your stamina increases, the same activity will feel easier, and your RPE score will gradually drop.

Tracking Strength: Measuring Your Power

Strength isn't just about lifting heavy weights—it's about the ability to perform movements that require power and stability. Without a gym, you might think it's difficult to track strength progress, but there are several effective ways to measure your progress using bodyweight exercises or minimal equipment.

1. Reps and Sets:

The most straightforward method of tracking strength is counting how many repetitions of an exercise you can complete with good form. For example, if you start by doing 10 push-ups, try adding one or two more each week. Record your sets, and note if you're able to do more or if you can do a particular exercise with less fatigue.

2. Progressive Variations:

Once you can perform an exercise with ease, it's time to move to a more challenging variation. For instance, if you're doing regular push-ups, progress to decline push-ups, clapping push-ups, or one-arm push-ups. Similarly, for squats, try adding a jump or holding a weight. Tracking your strength is all about noting when you're able to progress to more advanced variations, and it's a sign of your increasing power.

3. Form and Technique:

Strength doesn't just come from how many reps you do, but how well you do them. It's important to focus on proper technique, as it ensures you're building functional strength and not risking injury. Keep a log of how your form improves over time. For example, when you first start, you might need to do push-ups on your knees or practice squats in front of a mirror to make sure your knees don't collapse inward. Tracking the gradual improvement in form can give you a sense of accomplishment, even before increasing the number of reps.

Flexibility: Tracking Mobility Gains

Flexibility isn't just about being able to touch your toes—it's about the ability of your muscles and joints to move through a full range of motion. Flexibility helps prevent injuries, improves posture, and allows you to perform functional movements with ease. Tracking your flexibility progress is a great way to see measurable improvements in mobility and range of motion.

1. Simple Flexibility Tests:

One of the easiest ways to track flexibility is by performing simple tests at home. For instance, you can measure how far you can reach with your hands in a standing hamstring stretch or how far you can bend your knees while seated. Over time, you'll notice that you can reach further or bend deeper, which signifies improved flexibility.

2. Progressive Stretching Routines:

Creating a stretching or mobility routine can help you see consistent improvements. Incorporate stretches for key muscle groups—such as hamstrings, hip flexors, lower back, and shoulders—into your routine. Record your flexibility at the start of each session. After a few weeks of consistent practice, you should begin to see progress. You can track this through how much longer you hold a stretch or how much deeper you can go.

3. Yoga and Pilates Practice:

Yoga and Pilates are excellent ways to track flexibility progress since both practices emphasize mobility and flexibility alongside strength. Tracking your ability to hold certain poses, such as downward dog or pigeon pose, can show you tangible results.

Journaling and Habit Tracking: A Personal Record

One of the most powerful ways to track progress without feeling overwhelmed is to keep a simple fitness journal or habit tracker. Journaling helps create a mental connection to your fitness routine and allows you to look back at how far you've come. A fitness journal doesn't need to be anything fancy—just a notebook where you jot down key details of your workouts and progress.

1. Recording Workouts:

Write down what exercises you did, how many sets and reps, and any notes about how the workout felt. Tracking how you felt—whether energized or fatigued—helps you spot patterns in your body's responses and adjust accordingly.

2. Daily Habits:

For a holistic view, track daily habits such as your sleep, diet, and water intake. You may be surprised to see how these factors influence your fitness progress. A simple habit tracker can help you check off the days you meet your goals, creating a sense of accomplishment.

The Role of Wearable Tech

Wearable fitness trackers—such as Fitbit, Garmin, or Apple Watch—have become invaluable tools for tracking progress. These devices can track a variety of metrics like heart rate, steps, calories burned, sleep patterns, and even stress levels. Wearable tech is an excellent way to gain insights into your overall health, providing real-time data to help you make informed decisions.

1. Heart Rate and Recovery:

Many fitness trackers monitor heart rate during exercise and recovery periods. As your cardiovascular fitness improves, you'll notice that your heart rate drops quicker after exertion, signaling better stamina and recovery.

2. Sleep and Activity Patterns:

Sleep plays a critical role in recovery and overall fitness. A wearable can track your sleep patterns, providing feedback on how your rest correlates with your performance during workouts. Additionally, tracking your step count and general activity levels throughout the day helps you stay mindful of how much you're moving outside formal workouts.

Conclusion: Progress Over Perfection

Tracking your fitness journey without overwhelming yourself is about finding a balance. It's not about obsessively measuring every metric but rather creating a system that works for you and gives you tangible evidence of your improvements. By tracking stamina, strength, and flexibility, journaling your efforts, and using wearable tech as a helpful tool, you can maintain motivation and see the results of your hard work—without the stress of trying to keep up with unrealistic standards. Progress, after all, is personal. Celebrate each milestone, no matter how small, and remember that fitness is a lifelong journey, not a destination.

CHAPTER 19

OVERCOMING PLATEAUS

In the pursuit of fitness, progress can often feel like a steady climb, with visible improvements week after week. But what happens when that climb starts to level off? What do you do when the scale stops moving, your strength plateaus, or your endurance seems stuck at a certain point? This is the frustrating reality of fitness plateaus—those periods where it feels like you're putting in the work but seeing little to no results.

The good news is that plateaus are normal. Everyone experiences them at some point. The better news is that with the right strategies, you can break through these stagnation points and continue your fitness journey with renewed vigor. In this chapter, we'll explore how to overcome plateaus by mixing up your routine, adding new challenges, and applying proven techniques that keep you progressing.

Understanding Why Plateaus Happen

Before diving into strategies to overcome plateaus, it's important to understand why they occur in the first place. A plateau happens when your body adapts to your current routine. As you get fitter, your muscles and cardiovascular system become more efficient at handling the demands you place on them. This means that the same exercises, intensity, and frequency won't challenge your body in the same way they once did. The body no longer sees the need to adapt or improve.

Additionally, plateaus can also result from mental fatigue. When you've been doing the same routine for weeks or months, it can become monotonous. This mental boredom can affect motivation and make it harder to push through.

But rest assured, stagnation is a natural part of the process. The key is not to let it derail your progress. Instead, use it as an opportunity to grow stronger, more resilient, and more creative in your approach to fitness.

1. Change Your Routine: The Power of Variety

The quickest way to break through a plateau is to change things up. Your muscles—and mind—thrive on variety. Repetition leads to adaptation, but it can also lead to boredom, so introducing new elements to your workout is essential for continued progress.

Switch Up Your Exercises

If you've been doing the same exercises for a while, your body has likely adapted to them. For example, if you're used to doing 30-minute jogs every morning, your body has become efficient at this activity. You might not be burning as many calories, or you may not be improving your endurance at the same rate anymore. To push through this, it's important to introduce new exercises that challenge your body in different ways.

- Try New Types of Cardio: Instead of running, experiment with cycling, swimming, rowing, or jumping rope. These activities work different muscles and provide new cardiovascular challenges.

- Incorporate Different Strength Exercises: If you've been focusing primarily on squats, push-ups, and lunges, try variations like Bulgarian split squats, decline push-ups, or resistance band exercises. Challenge your muscles by switching between bodyweight exercises and using household items (e.g., water bottles, bags of rice) for resistance.

- Change Your Focus: If you've primarily focused on strength training, shift your attention to flexibility or balance. Practices like yoga or Pilates will engage your core in ways that traditional exercises might not.

Change Your Reps, Sets, and Rest Periods

Sometimes the change you need isn't in the exercise itself, but in the structure of your workout. If you've been sticking to the same number of reps and sets, it's time to shake things up:

- Increase or Decrease Your Reps: Try going for higher reps with lower weights (for endurance) or fewer reps with higher weights (for strength). The change in intensity forces your body to adapt in new ways.

- Vary Your Rest Periods: Shortening or lengthening your rest periods can make a huge difference in the effectiveness of your workout. Try training with minimal rest between sets to increase endurance, or give yourself longer rest periods to push heavier weights for strength.

- Try Supersets or Circuit Training: Instead of completing all sets for one exercise before moving on, try combining exercises into supersets or circuit-style training. This increases workout intensity and targets multiple muscle groups at once, helping you break through that plateau.

2. Introduce New Challenges: Take It Up a Notch

Once you've introduced some variety to your routine, it's time to start pushing your limits by introducing new challenges. This can involve increasing intensity, adding complexity, or setting new performance goals. By challenging yourself, you force your body to keep adapting.

Progressive Overload

Progressive overload is the foundation of strength training and muscle growth. It means gradually increasing the intensity of your workouts to continue challenging your muscles. You can apply progressive overload in several ways:

- Increase Resistance: Add weight to your bodyweight exercises (using dumbbells, resistance bands, or household objects) to continue building strength.

- Increase Volume: Increase the number of sets or reps you're doing for each exercise.

- Increase Intensity: Perform exercises more quickly, add plyometric (explosive) movements, or decrease rest time between sets to raise the intensity of your workout.

Focus on Skill Development

Sometimes, progressing doesn't just mean lifting heavier weights or running longer distances—it's about mastering new skills. For example:

- Mastering Yoga Poses: If you've been practicing yoga for a while, try moving into more advanced poses like handstands or arm balances.

- Learning to Sprint: If you're a runner, focus on improving your sprinting speed or form. Interval training with sprints can break through a plateau in endurance.

- Perfecting Your Push-Up Technique: If you've been doing regular push-ups for a while, challenge yourself to progress to more advanced push-up variations, like one-arm push-ups or clapping push-ups.

3. Mentally Challenge Yourself: The Power of Mindset

Physical stagnation often has a mental component as well. If you're stuck in a rut, it's essential to address the mental barriers that might be holding you back. Setting new goals, focusing on your "why," and shifting your mindset are key factors in overcoming plateaus.

- Set New Goals: If you've been fixated on a specific goal (like losing weight or running a certain distance), change your focus. Set performance-based goals instead—such as mastering a new exercise, completing a more challenging workout, or increasing your strength by a certain amount.

- Find Accountability: Whether through a workout buddy, a fitness community, or an app, accountability can provide the motivation you need to push through stagnation.

- Celebrate Small Wins: Sometimes, the breakthrough comes when you stop obsessing over the "big picture." Celebrate small victories, like doing an extra rep, holding a plank for a few seconds longer, or pushing yourself through a tough workout.

4. Rest and Recovery: Don't Forget the Importance of Balance

As you intensify your workouts, it's equally important to ensure you're giving your body enough time to rest and recover. Overtraining can lead to burnout and even further plateaus. Rest is just as vital as the effort you put into your workouts.

- Listen to Your Body: If you feel fatigued or notice a decline in performance, it may be time to incorporate more rest days or active recovery (e.g., light yoga or walking).

- Get Quality Sleep: Recovery happens during sleep. Ensure you're getting enough rest to allow your muscles to repair and grow stronger.

Conclusion: Keep Pushing Forward

Plateaus are an inevitable part of any fitness journey, but they don't have to be permanent. By introducing variety, increasing the challenge, and focusing on mental and physical recovery, you can continue to make progress and push beyond your limits. Fitness is about more than just breaking through barriers—it's about creating a sustainable, enjoyable journey toward becoming the best version of yourself.

CHAPTER 20

SUSTAINABLE FITNESS FOR LIFE

Fitness isn't a destination; it's a lifelong journey. The most successful fitness routines aren't the ones that promise rapid transformations but the ones that become so ingrained in your daily life that they feel like second nature. Sustainable fitness is about creating habits that not only last but thrive in your everyday routine, making health and movement an essential part of who you are.

In this chapter, we'll explore how to cultivate habits that stick, find joy in the process of movement, and weave fitness seamlessly into your lifestyle. By the end of this chapter, you'll have the tools to embrace fitness for life, making it an enduring, enjoyable part of your everyday routine.

1. Cultivating Habits That Stick

When it comes to fitness, consistency is key. The challenge isn't in starting; it's in maintaining. The key to long-term fitness success lies in the creation of sustainable habits—small, incremental steps that you can sustain over the long term without burning out.

Start Small, Start Smart

One of the most common pitfalls people face when attempting to adopt a fitness routine is trying to do too much too quickly. Setting overly ambitious goals right away is a recipe for frustration and burnout. Instead, start small. Choose an activity you can easily commit to—whether it's a daily 10-minute stretch session, a brisk 15-minute walk, or a simple bodyweight workout. The goal is to create a habit that doesn't feel daunting.

For example, instead of committing to an hour of exercise every day, set a goal to be active for 20 minutes three times a week. Once you consistently hit that target, gradually increase the intensity or duration of your sessions. Small wins lead to big changes, and each small success builds confidence and reinforces your commitment.

Routine Is Your Friend

The power of habit lies in routine. One of the best ways to make fitness stick is to integrate it into your daily schedule at a set time. Whether it's in the morning before work, during your lunch break, or in the evening after dinner, creating a predictable time for movement ensures that fitness becomes as regular as brushing your teeth.

Consistency doesn't mean rigidity. Life happens, and flexibility is important. If you miss a workout, don't let it derail your entire week. Simply adjust, and get back on track the next day. What matters most is that fitness becomes a non-negotiable part of your lifestyle over time.

2. Finding Joy in Movement

The best fitness routines aren't just about achieving aesthetic goals or following trends—they're about discovering what makes you feel good. Movement should be enjoyable, not a chore. The more joy you find in exercise, the more likely it is that you'll stick with it. The key is to experiment with different forms of movement and find what brings you joy.

Rediscover Play

As children, movement was second nature. We ran, jumped, and played without worrying about whether we were "exercising." As adults, we often forget the fun of movement. To build a lifelong love of fitness, try to rediscover that playful spirit. Go for a walk in the park, play a sport with friends, or join a dance class. Activities like hiking, cycling, or swimming not only engage the body but also bring a sense of freedom and enjoyment that traditional gym workouts often lack.

Sometimes, fitness can be disguised as play. Jumping rope, playing tag with your kids, or even climbing trees— these activities engage the body in functional ways while keeping you entertained. The joy in these activities often comes from being immersed in the moment, free from the pressure of performance or results. Make movement fun again, and it will become something you look forward to.

Find Your Flow

Flow is that magical state where you're completely absorbed in what you're doing. You lose track of time and feel a sense of ease and accomplishment. When it comes to fitness, finding activities that allow you to enter this flow state is crucial. Whether it's yoga, running, cycling, or even a long walk, the idea is to find a movement pattern that feels natural and effortless to you.

For example, if you enjoy running, try exploring different trails in your area, taking in the scenery as you run. If yoga is your thing, focus less on the perfect pose and more on how your body feels as you move from one posture to the next. The key to lasting enjoyment is not forcing yourself into an exercise you dread but allowing your body to naturally gravitate toward activities that make you feel good.

Challenge Yourself, but Don't Overwhelm Yourself

It's important to keep pushing your limits, but fitness should not feel like an endless cycle of struggle. If you make progress in your fitness routine, celebrate those wins. Don't fall into the trap of constantly comparing yourself to others. Fitness is a personal journey, and you're the only one who can measure your progress.

Setting achievable challenges can also help you maintain a sense of motivation and accomplishment. If you've mastered 10 push-ups, set a goal for 15. If you can walk for 20 minutes, aim to walk for 30. By continuously setting attainable goals, you ensure a sense of growth without overwhelming yourself with unattainable expectations.

3. Making Fitness a Natural Part of Your Day

To make fitness sustainable, it has to blend seamlessly into your daily life. It shouldn't be something that feels like an "extra" but rather an integral part of your routine. Here's how you can make fitness part of your everyday life.

Movement Throughout the Day

One of the easiest ways to stay active without committing to a structured workout is to incorporate movement into your daily activities. Take the stairs instead of the elevator, walk or bike instead of driving, stretch or stand every 30 minutes if you work at a desk. Little changes like these can accumulate throughout the day to add up to significant benefits. It's not about finding time for fitness but rather making time for movement within your existing schedule.

Active Recovery

You don't need to work out intensely every day. In fact, rest and recovery are as important as the workouts themselves. Active recovery days are when you engage in low-intensity activities like walking, yoga, or light stretching. These help maintain movement while allowing your body to recover and rebuild. It's these lighter, less intense days that allow fitness to be sustainable in the long term, ensuring you don't burn out.

Set Realistic Expectations

Life can be busy, and fitness won't always be at the top of your priority list. That's okay. Set realistic expectations for yourself. Don't expect to work out every day or to make every session perfect. What's important is that you keep showing up, even when life gets in the way.

Conclusion: Fitness for Life

Sustainable fitness is all about creating a lifestyle that incorporates movement as naturally as breathing. It's about building habits that serve your body and mind, finding joy in movement, and integrating fitness into every part of your life. With the right mindset and the willingness to experiment, fitness can become a lifelong journey that enriches your life in countless ways.

So, take a deep breath, step outside, and remember: fitness isn't about the gym. It's about living a life full of movement, joy, and wellness—one small step at a time.

The Lifelong Journey Ahead

As we reach the end of this book, remember that the real work begins when you close its pages and step back into the world. Fitness is not something you achieve in a few weeks or months—it's a lifelong journey, and every day offers an opportunity to move forward, to grow stronger, and to feel better, no matter where you are or what stage you're at.

There will be days when motivation wanes, when life gets busy, or when you feel tempted to skip that workout or choose convenience over health. But in those moments, remember that fitness isn't a destination—it's a way of living. It's about finding joy in movement, embracing your body's power, and continuing to nurture your health in ways that feel authentic to you.

You don't need a gym to stay fit. You have everything you need within you—your body, your curiosity, and your willingness to show up, even on the hard days. Whether it's through a morning walk, a fun dance class, or a simple stretch before bed, every movement counts, and every effort is progress.

As you move forward, don't be afraid to adapt, experiment, and most importantly, enjoy the process. Make fitness a natural part of your daily routine, and trust that, over time, it will transform not just your body, but your life.

So, go ahead. Take that first step, or perhaps the next one. Your fitness journey is uniquely yours, and the road ahead is full of possibility. Embrace it with patience, enthusiasm, and the belief that the best version of yourself is a lifelong work in progress.

Here's to a life of movement, strength, and wellness— one step at a time.

Thank you for Reading The Book.

www.ingramcontent.com/pod-product-compliance
Lightning Source LLC
Chambersburg PA
CBHW061040250726
48653CB00001B/186